Mother Nature's Guide
to Vibrant Beauty and Health

Other books by Myra Cameron:

HOME-STYLE MICROWAVE COOKING

THE G.N.C. GOURMET VITAMIN COOKBOOK

TREASURY OF HOME REMEDIES

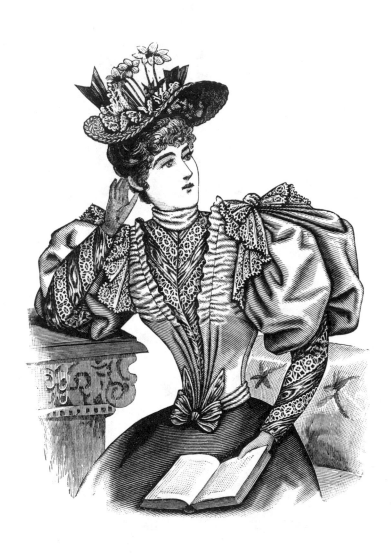

Mother Nature's
Guide
to Vibrant
Beauty and Health

Myra Cameron

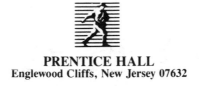

PRENTICE HALL
Englewood Cliffs, New Jersey 07632

Prentice-Hall International (UK) Limited, *London*
Prentice-Hall of Australia Pty. Limited, *Sydney*
Prentice-Hall Canada, Inc., *Toronto*
Prentice-Hall Hispanoamericana, S.A., *Mexico*
Prentice-Hall of India Private Limited, *New Delhi*
Prentice-Hall of Japan, Inc., *Tokyo*
Simon & Schuster Asia Pte. Ltd., *Singapore*
Editora Prentice-Hall do Brasil, Ltda., *Rio de Janeiro*

© 1990 *by*

PRENTICE-HALL, Inc.
Englewood Cliffs, NJ

This book is a reference work based on research. The opinions expressed herein
are not necessarily those of or endorsed by the publisher or author. The
directions stated in this book are in no way to be considered as a substitute for
consultation with a duly licensed doctor.

10   9   8   7   6   5   4   3

The art illustrations in this book originally appeared between 1892 and 1895
as advertisements in *The Delineator, A Journal of Fashion, Culture and Fine Arts*,
published by the Butterick Publishing Co. (Limited), London & New York.

Library of Congress Cataloging-in-Publication Data

Cameron, Myra.
  Mother Nature's guide to vibrant beauty and health / Myra Cameron.
    p.   cm.
  Includes bibliographical references.
  ISBN 0-13-603119-6   ISBN 0-13-601386-4 (pbk.)
  1. Skin—Care and hygiene.   2. Cosmetics.   3. Beauty, Personal.
4. Health.   I. Title.
RL87.C36   1990
646.7'2—dc20   89-25589
                                                                      CIP

ISBN 0-13-603119-6

ISBN 0-13-601386-4 (pbk)

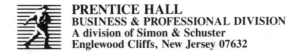
PRENTICE HALL
BUSINESS & PROFESSIONAL DIVISION
A division of Simon & Schuster
Englewood Cliffs, New Jersey 07632

Printed in the United States of America

How This Book Will Help You Look and Feel More Vibrant and Naturally Beautiful

Suppose there was a miracle product that could help clear up your skin problems, put a sparkle in your eyes, leave your hair looking thick and shining, and your body muscles lean and limber. Chances are you'd buy that product! In fact, Americans spend millions of dollars each year on fast-fix health cure-alls and commercial cosmetics that promise the world, but seldom deliver.

Yet, with a bit of help from you, and at practically no expense, radiant health and beauty can be yours. *Mother Nature's Guide to Vibrant Beauty and Health* offers a complete guide to genuine, do-it-yourself beauty care for women *and* men—without harsh, irritating chemicals or additives. In a world deluged by synthetics, reverting to nature's plan gives you safe and easy options for each of the many phases of beauty.

By combining centuries-old beauty secrets with up-to-date advice from modern dermatologists, nutritionists, physicians, and fitness experts, this *Guide* offers up-to-the-minute, time-tested secrets and all-natural remedies for tackling many of the beauty problems you thought were unsolvable.

Here are some of the many benefits you'll discover in this book:

- Tips on protecting your skin from seasonal changes
- Four everyday products from nature that safely remove makeup and clean skin

- An all-natural, updated recipe for making your own soap
- How to prepare your own skin-care products
- Do-it-yourself moisturizers for dewy-fresh skin
- How to give yourself an at-home facial with professional, salon-like results
- Natural masques from nature that rejuvenate and nourish your skin
- The safe way to eliminate blackheads and whiteheads
- All-natural treatments for clearing up skin discolorations
- Tips on nourishing maturing skin
- Herbs that enhance your bath
- How to play it safe in the sun—with natural remedies for relieving sunburn pain
- Natural remedies for correcting seven common foot problems
- 25 herbs that make effective mouth rinses
- Time-tested secrets for beautiful hands
- Nine soothing compresses and poultices for refreshing tired, irritated eyes
- Natural colorants to perk up your hair and shampoos you can make yourself
- How to snack nutritiously all day long
- Six-minute shape-up guide for toning and limbering
- Nine natural aids for combating stress

You'll find *Mother Nature's Guide to Vibrant Beauty and Health* to be an invaluable resource for healthful products and remedies. Radiant health and beauty *can* be yours—with the help of Mother Nature!

Preface

You can employ beauticians to glamorize your face with cosmetics, temporarily minimize wrinkles or bulges, and coif you with a wig. Playing Cinderella for an evening might be exciting; having genuine, do-it-yourself beauty is more rewarding. It reflects in your mirror at dawn, in the way you move, and in the eyes of your beholders. Clear skin, sparkling eyes, shining hair, and lithe muscles do not disappear when the clock strikes twelve. Beauty is the total you; it comes as a package deal. Nutrients you ingest, muscles you move, the way you cope with stress; all play a role in your beautiful image.

Along with her gift of a body, complete with a permanent covering of skin, Mother Nature has provided the wherewithall for its care. In a world deluged by synthetics, reverting to nature's plan may be wise because foods affect your exterior as well as your interior. The body's outer surface absorbs or reacts to substances with which it comes in contact, so why not feed your face (and your hands, feet, nails, and hair) with low-cost, healthful products instead of endangering them with expensive, chemically contrived beauty aids?

By correlating centuries-old beauty secrets with up-to-date advice from modern dermatologists, nutritionists, physicians, and fitness experts, *Mother Nature's Guide to Vibrant Beauty and Health* offers safe and easy options for each of the many phases of beauty. With its explicit step-by-step directions you can concoct your own facial masques, toners, and lotions. From the dietary guidelines you can create your individualized regimen of eating for beauty and energy. You can customize your personal muscle-toning and life-extending fitness program by selecting your choices from the exercises described. For your inner self there are mood-changing techniques to relieve tension or entice sleep; and, for your Prince Charming, there are "handsome" treatments and tips—men, too, have skin, nails, and hair.

Nurturing Mother Nature's gifts to make the most of your visible assets is not vanity. When you look and feel your best, you radiate an aura that attracts others and makes them receptive. Neglecting appearance and health isn't noble; it diminishes self-assurance, "turns off" those around you, and accelerates the aging process. The axiom "Pretty is as pretty does" still applies; it takes conscious effort to be beautiful. With this book as a guide, and a bit of your help, Mother Nature can be your fairy godmother—transforming you into a vibrantly lovely, full-time Cinderella. No matter what your age may be at this moment, *now* is the time to begin your transformation.

Contents

Section 1

Making the Most of Your Skin

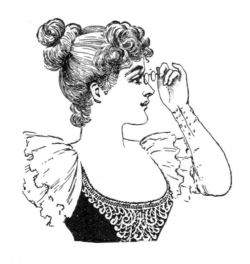

How to Have Beautifully Healthy Skin

You can hide your hair beneath a wig and wear a mu-mu to conceal figure faults, but until veiled hats come back in style, your face is up front for everyone to see—and even professional makeup can only temporarily mask skin that has been ignored or mistreated. The men in your life can also reap the benefits of skin pampering. Fifteen years ago, the few men who entered prestigious Madison Avenue skin-care salons sidled through rear entrances. Today, conscious of the importance of outward appearance in business and social life, over half the salon clients are men.

Skin: The Vital Statistics

MIRACLE COVERING SUBSTANCE

Lightweight & Flexible—conforms to any shape
Elastic—will expand up to 40 times its original size
Waterproof—forms a two-way barrier between fluids
Self-mending—reseals itself if burned, cut, or punctured
Washable & Durable—one coating lasts a lifetime

The response to the above advertisement would be a line of prospective purchasers encircling the globe. Most of life's best sensations pass through the outer covering, yet skin is not for sale, it is a miraculous gift from Mother Nature. Even its vital statistics are fascinating: skin varies in thickness from 1/50 of an inch over the eardrums to 1/4 of an inch on the soles of the feet. The 15 to 20 square feet of skin required to encase an adult weighs approximately 20 pounds. It protects us from environmental pollutants, contains and early-warning-device to inform us of impending danger from extreme heat or cold, and is an automatic thermostat that helps regulate body temperature.

There is more to skin than meets the eye. The epidermis, the surface we see, is composed primarily of dead skin and melanocytes (pigment cells) performing their protective duties while waiting to be sloughed off. Beneath the epidermis lies the dermis, a veritable beehive of activity. Within it flourish collagen and elastin (the fibrous supportive system), hair follicles, tiny blood vessels, and the sebaceous glands which supply fluids to fuel and lubricate the skin. A resilient subcutaneous layer below the dermis further supports the skin and cushions internal bones and organs from shock. The amount of sebum (a waxy-oily substance) exuded by the sebaceous glands is largely responsible for the type of skin we have.

Dry, *oily*, or *normal* are the stereotyped labels for skin. *Combination* or *mosaic* is how most facial skin really is, and it usually has a "T-zone" of oiliness across the forehead and down the nose, with dryness on the cheeks. Whatever your skin type may be at the moment, it is subject to change with very little notice.

Tips on Protecting Your Skin from Seasonal Changes

Like the exterior walls of your home, your skin is your body's shelter. Exposed to the elements and to your physical environment, it has an outer as well as an inner life. It copes with summer heat and wintry chill; industrial fumes, smoke, fog, smog, dust, and soot; plus sudden fluctuations in temperature caused by air conditioning and forced-air heating.

How to winterize your skin

Winter is beauty's enemy. Outdoor cold and wind attack your skin, indoor heat robs it of moisture. Dry skin suffers more than oily skin, but every type of skin benefits from these defensive measures:

- Tone and moisturize (see Chapters 3 and 4) after each cleansing to preserve and replenish the moisture in your skin. Use a moisturizing night nourisher every evening. Apply a daytime moisturizer around your eyes and on dry-skin areas each morning.

- Add skin-pampering ingredients to your bath (see Chapter 8) to prevent allover dryness.

- Wait 30 minutes after bathing, or washing your face, before going out into frigid air. Splash your face with cool water when you come back inside. Extreme temperature changes can burst capillaries near the skin's surface.

- Moisturize indoor air by plugging in a humidifier, by placing a damp towel or a pan of water near the heat source, or by surrounding yourself with growing plants.

How to summerize your skin

Although summer is kinder than winter to dry skin, it accentuates oily-skin problems and necessitates a different skin-protective campaign.

- Give your face an extra cleansing each day and always clean your face after strenuous activity. Warm weather means more active oil glands. Perspiration makes dirt cling to your skin.

- Use a "light" night cream and daytime moisturizer. Smooth on only a few drops to compensate for the extra washing and perspiring that remove the skin's invisible shield. Use additional moisturizer when you travel by plane; pressurized air is excessively dry.

- Watch out for the sun; too much of it makes skin lined, leathery, and old before its time.

Seven Ways To Promote—and Prolong—a More Youthful Appearance

Skin is more than just a covering; it is a barometer that registers the state of our health and reveals the story of our lives. The decline and fall of our epidermis does not become apparent until we pass the 30-year milestone, but it actually begins at birth. Our "perfect" baby skin alters with puberty; undergoes more variations from hormonal fluctuations during menstrual cycles, pregnancy, and menopause; then gradually becomes thinner, drier, and less supple as cell functions slow with age.

Chronologically, we all grow old at the same rate. Visibly, we age at an individual pace—and it's never too early or late to start improving your skin.

Life expectancy is now double what it was a few centuries ago, more than triple the original design which anticipated death shortly after the conclusion of a short span of reproductive ability. Evolutionary alterations to delay the biological processes of approaching old age are a future probability. Meanwhile, if we are to save our twentieth-century faces, it's up to us to assist Mother Nature. Prolonging a youthful appearance by keeping up with changes as they occur is easier than rejuvenating the ravages wrought by Father Time.

Acne (see Chapter 6) attacks more boys than girls during the teenage years, but besets more women than men because oral contraceptives, menstruation, and menopause cause hormone levels to surge and wane.

Pregnancy profoundly affects the skin. For the first five months, increased estrogen production suppresses the natural skin-lubricating oils to make skin drier than normal. Use a mild, nondetergent cleanser, a nourishing moisturizer during the day, and apply a rich night cream before retiring. During the latter half of pregnancy, an upswing of progesterone hormones may make skin oilier and more subject to blemishes. Cleanse your skin thoroughly, use an astringent toner, cut back on your moisturizing routine, and guard against the brown splotches of a pregnancy mask by applying a potent sunscreen before venturing forth in daylight.

While waiting for the fountain of perpetual youth to be discovered, you can prolong a youthful appearance if you:

1. Incorporate more moisturizing in your daily-care routine to compensate for the reduced activity of sweat and sebaceous glands, which causes gradual drying and thinning of the skin.

2. Forestall photoaging by applying a sunscreen and sunning safely (see Chapter 9).

3. Exercise regularly to maintain the blood circulation essential for bringing nourishment to the dermal vessels and for carrying off wastes from the skin. Reclining on a slantboard also improves circulation, and the "downhill" position negates some of the sags, wrinkles, and droops attributable to gravity.

4. Deliberately relax away tension (see Chapter 17) to help prevent "expression lines" in your face, and other stress-related skin problems.

5. Get sufficient sleep so your skin can receive its fresh supplies of oxygen and nutrients.

6. Keep your weight fairly constant to avoid the saggy wrinkles that can develop when yo-yo dieting leaves stretched skin without underlying support.

7. Eat a well-balanced diet to help maintain and rebuild the supportive tissues, and to preserve the visible surface.

Inside-out Care for a Flawless Complexion

How to care for your skin from the inside

What you eat, or don't eat, is revealed by your skin: nutrients absorbed into the bloodstream nourish it through loops of capillaries close to the surface. Radiantly healthy skin is one of the dividends of eating a nutritionally balanced diet (see Chapter 15), taking supplements when needed, and drinking six to eight glasses of water each day. Fruit and vegetable juices or herbal teas may be substituted for some of the water. Alcoholic drinks and caffeine-containing beverages, (regular coffee, tea, some herbal teas, many soft drinks) act as mild diuretics to dehydrate your system, so they shouldn't be counted on for filling the quota. Drinking two glasses of barley juice each day is credited with maintaining the flawless complexions of British royalty.[102]

Here's how to prepare your own *Royal Barley Juice*: Simmer 1/4 cup pearl barley in 5 cups of water in a covered saucepan for 1 hour. Squeeze 1 lemon and 3 oranges, reserve the juice, add the rinds to the saucepan, and let stand until cool. Strain the liquid into a pitcher, stir in the reserved juice plus honey to taste, then store in the refrigerator.

PROTEIN: Skin is predominantly protein, requires a daily supply from the foods you eat because protein molecules are not absorbed through the epidermis into underlying tissues,[45] and registers a deficiency by becoming slack and loose. Collagen-containing protein foods (avocados, brewer's yeast, dried legumes, nuts, sesame and sunflower seeds, whole grain cereals) help prevent and smooth out wrinkles. Other protein foods (fish, meats, poultry, eggs, dairy products, vegetable proteins) help your body equalize the balance between new and dying cells.

FATS AND OILS: The unsaturated fats in vegetable oils assist assimilation of fat-soluble vitamins A, D, and E; contribute to your own natural oils to give your skin a sheen, plump out fine lines, and create the fresh-faced look of youth. One or two tablespoons a day can be used as salad dressing or whizzed in the blender with milk, fruit or vegetable drinks.

FRUITS, VEGETABLES, AND FIBER: In addition to varying amounts of protein and the complex carbohydrates needed for energy, fruits and vegetables provide the fiber (grandmother called it roughage) to keep you vibrantly beautiful and healthy by flushing toxins out of your body and avoiding constipation. If you run short, a tablespoon of miller's bran each day should help. Fresh, raw foods also contain enzymes that act as the body's housekeepers to keep the bloodstream clear, and, cooked or uncooked, fruits and vegetables offer an appetizing supply of vitamins and minerals necessary for skin health.

VITAMINS AND MINERALS: Overindulging in anything, particularly fat-soluble vitamins A, D, and E, can be dangerous. Some of the following supplements may be in order, however, because individual requirements may be higher than the official RDA (recommended dietary allowance), and because eating sufficient quantities of their natural food sources (see the Vitamin and Mineral Chart) is either impractical (76 oranges equal 500 milligrams of vitamin C) or would lead to unwanted weight gain.

- Vitamin A is used to preserve a smooth skin texture, prevent dryness, and avoid blemishes or hasten their healing.

- B Vitamins are vital for clear, luminous skin. Only about 1 percent of the water-soluble, must-be-replenished-daily B complex ingested is routed to the skin, and, because they function interactively, a deficiency of any of the Bs can cause skin problems. Insufficiencies may make themselves apparent by inflamed fissures at the angles of the nose and mouth, scaly lips, premature wrinkles, or by other skin disturbances.[92] Studies show that 40 percent of dermatitis sufferers lack B vitamins.[32]

- Vitamin C, in conjunction with protein, is necessary for the production of collagen—the glue that holds us and our skin together and circumvents sags or wrinkles. Combined with bioflavinoids, vitamin C helps prevent the pigment clumping that the sun turns into "age spots," and strengthens capillaries to avoid easy bruising or the tiny hemorrhages that become spider veins. Vitamin C also helps the oil-secreting glands function properly to keep the skin from drying out. If you're a cigarette smoker, supplemental C is advisable. Cigarettes devour at least 500 milligrams per pack, or up to 5,000 milligrams, according to Irwin Stone, author of *Vitamin C Against Disease* (Grosset & Dunlap, 1972).

- Vitamin E, necessary for healthy, moist skin, is an antioxidant present in vegetable oils; yet additional amounts of E are required to prevent the E in the oils from oxidation within the body. Biochemical research has demonstrated that large doses of vitamin E double healthy cell reproduction to slow the aging process and forestall premature wrinkling.[19] *Caution:* If you have diabetes, high blood pressure, or an overactive thyroid, check with your physician before taking supplemental E.

- Minerals all contribute to our beauty and well-being. Two of the most essential for skin care are

   Copper—important for the production of skin pigment, and for the prevention of blotches under the skin from ruptured blood vessels. It also cooperates with other nutrients to preserve the integrity of the elastic-like fibers supporting the skin.

   Zinc—aids in the formation of collagen, helps prevent dry skin and stretch marks, and promotes blemish healing. Without enough zinc a deficiency of Vitamin A can occur even though the intake of that vitamin appears adequate.

How to care for your skin from the outside

If you treat your skin with tenderness, it will respond with finely textured dewy freshness. If you neglect your skin, overexpose it to the sun, abuse it with harsh soaps and abrasive cleansers, irritate it with stinging astringents, or suffocate it with leftover makeup and heavy creams, it will retaliate by flaking away, erupting in bumps, developing splotches, bursting its capillaries, and wrinkling prematurely. Caring for your skin gently and consistently is the key to extending its youthful appearance.

The once-held belief that skin is an impenetrable barrier turns out to be a myth. Laboratory studies reported in *Health* (May, 1986) indicate that many substances are absorbed through the skin, reach the bloodstream, and are transported throughout the body. Iodine, for instance, can be detected in the urine shortly after it is applied to unbroken skin. Dermatologists now agree that *everything* permeates to some extent. According to Dr. Peter M. Elias of the University of California at San Francisco, the degree of absorption varies with the substance and the body area. The face is ten times more permeable than any other part of the body, with water and alcohol solutions (colognes and astringents) penetrating most easily; water and oil-based emulsions (moisturizers) next; and little absorption from sunscreens or the brief contact of cleansers. "Feeding your face" is more than just a witticism. Tests conducted at Purdue University show that natural foods benefit the skin when used cosmetically (see

Chapter 3); they are not only harmless, they are often more effective than chemical-containing commercial cosmetics.[132]

Skin's response to a program of systematic care is almost instantaneous, and, as young cells migrate up through the dermis to replace dead cells sloughed off the surface in a constant process of self-renewal, we have a "new" face every 28 days. "Regimen" sounds intimidating. A daily routine of skin care requires no more than ten minutes, and requires only three simple steps—cleanse, tone, and moisturize—each evening and morning.

Night care

1. Cleanse. Remove any makeup with cleansing cream or a natural makeup remover. Wash with mild soap or other cleanser, rinse, and pat dry.
2. Tone. Apply an acid-containing solution to restore the pH balance and protective shield. For dry skin, use a mild freshener-toner. For oily skin, use an astringent preparation.
3. Moisturize. Splash on cool water or mist with a spray bottle. Blot, but do not dry completely—moisturizer magic relies more on retaining moisture than in providing it—then smooth on a few drops of your moisturizer.

Day care

1. Cleanse lightly to remove nighttime accumulations, refresh your face with a few splashes of water, and pat dry.
2. Tone by applying a freshener or astringent.
3. Moisturize around your eyes. If your face is excessively dry, mist or splash with water, blot, then lightly cover with moisturizer.

❧ 2 ❧

Tips on Safely &
Gently Cleansing
Your Face & Throat

Clean skin is essential for both beauty and health; we breathe through skin pores as well as through nose and mouth. Horror tales of circus performers perishing after being coated with gilt paint do not create a precedent for sudden death following one night of sleeping with the day's accumulation of perspiration and pollutants. However, habitually retiring uncleansed may damage more than your pillow case: dry skin areas can become more sensitive; normal or oily skin can develop enlarged pores, blackheads, blemishes or similar unpleasantries; and your skin may lose its luminosity.

Beyond the Kitchen: Four Everyday Products from Nature That Safely Remove Makeup and Cleanse Skin

If you wear makeup, getting all of it off your face is the first stage of cleansing. Commercial creams or lotions are not the only options; Mother Nature offers a full line you can share with your favorite male if he makes "on camera" appearances. (Stage makeup is harsher than the department store products, he should allow several hours between shaving and its application.)

1. Mayonnaise. Bottled or homemade (see Glossary for recipe), mayonnaise is surprisingly effective. Smooth on, tissue off, or remove with a damp washcloth.
2. Milk. Shake 2 tablespoons of warm, whole milk with 1/4 teaspoon oil. Apply with a cotton ball, then tissue off.
3. Vegetable oil. Dip a cotton ball into your favorite salad oil, swish over eyes and lips, and gently wipe off. Saturate another cotton ball to coat your face, wait a few seconds for it to permeate, then remove it with a tissue or damp cloth.
4. White vegetable shortening. This can be smoothed on like a cleansing cream, allowed to remain for a minute, then removed with gentle, upward sweeps of a tissue or damp washcloth.

An All-natural, Updated Approach to Making Your Own Soap

Even if you don't wear makeup, the day's conglomeration of contaminants should be removed. What should you use to cleanse your face? Soap (which emulsifies the particulates and skin oils lurking on the surface) and water (which can't go it alone but is essential for rinsing) are the most popular and most efficient of many choices. The soap-making art has advanced considerably in the 2,000 years since the Romans boiled goat tallow with wood ashes to duplicate the foamy suds that billowed up when rain fell on the charred remains of sacrificed animals. Today's detergent-deodorant soaps and those containing abrasive granules are too harsh for facial use, but there are superfatted and cold-cream beauty bars scented with perfume, liquid soaps in pump dispensers, transparent soaps filled with glycerin, floating soaps filled with air, pure castile cakes that smell like soap, and do-it-yourself options.

Homemade natural glycerin beauty bars

This homemade soap contains a natural glycerin (formed by the chemical reaction of fat and caustic but removed from commercial products for separate sale), so much skin-softening oil it is low-sudsing, and you can manufacture 10 pounds of it without butchering a beast or building an outdoor fire. The equipment required is minimal: an 8-quart enamel or nonmetal cooking pot; an immersible thermometer that registers as low as 90 degrees Farenheit; a long-handled wooden spoon; cheesecloth, muslin or plastic wrap; and three 9-by-14-inch glass baking pans or cardboard boxes, or an array of custard cups. The ingredients can be obtained from your grocery or drugstore.

5 pounds pure lard

2 cups hot water (chlorine free)

2 cups olive oil

6 cups cold water (chlorine free)

1 twelve-ounce can 100% lye

3/4 cup almond or coconut oil

1 tablespoon tincture of benzoin

optional perfume: 2 tablespoons oil of lavender, lemon, lemon grass, musk, or other fragrance

Place the lard and hot water in the cooking container and heat until the fat is melted. Remove from heat, stir in the olive oil, and let stand until the temperature drops to 100 degrees. Pour the cold water into a 4-quart glass bowl, slowly stir in the lye with the wooden spoon. Let cool to 90 degrees. Gradually stir the lye-water into the melted fat, stirring until it is thick and creamy, then beat in the almond or coconut oil, benzoin, and perfume (if used).

Line the pans, boxes, or dishes with plastic wrap or wet cloth. Ladle in your "soap" to a depth of about 1-1/8 inch. Let stand for 8 to 16 hours (until firm), remove from the containers and cut into bars. "Cure" for at least two weeks by layering the bars in a carton on sheets of cardboard.

Oatmeal beauty bars

Grind 2 cups of oatmeal in an electric blender or food processor. After half the creamy soap has been transferred to its mold, beat the oatmeal into the remainder and proceed as with the natural glycerin bars.

"Bonus Bar" is Richard's name for this oatmeal variation. He had been skeptical about Sally's "kettleful of grease" ever turning into soap, had even questioned the project's necessity. "Why don't you just buy some? Stores do sell soap," he said, "ready-made, cut into bars and everything." However, Sally's skin felt so soft after a few days of using her homemade beauty bar that Richard agreed to experiment—just in case it might smooth up his flaky forehead. It did—so successfully that he volunteered to assist with cooking up the next batch of soap!

Three No-Fuss Ways to Improve Store-bought Soap

For "no curing required" soaps, try one of these mixtures. The bars have a base of two 4-ounce cakes of white castile soap, grated by hand or in a food processor.

SCENTED SOAP FOR SOFTENING AND WHITENING: Melt the grated soap in the top of the double boiler with 1/4 cup alcohol *or* strained, fresh lemon juice. Stir in 1/4 cup of your favorite cologne and 1 tablespoon glycerin before transferring to a foil-lined loaf pan to harden.

SKIN-SOFTENING OATMEAL SOAP: Combine the grated soap with 1/4 cup almond oil in the top of a double boiler. Heat until the soap melts, then stir in 1-1/3 cups uncooked oatmeal (pulverized in an electric blender, if desired). Transfer to a foil-lined loaf pan to harden.

ALMOND-MEAL SOFTSOAP: This mild, liquid soap was a favored complexion cleanser during the 1800s. For easy preparation with modern equipment, blend 2 tablespoons almond meal with 1/2 cup rose water and one-fourth of a 4-ounce bar of unscented castile soap grated into a food processor. Process with a cutting blade while gradually adding more rose water until the mixture looks like milk. (A hand grater, mixing bowl, and rotary egg beater may be used for nonelectric preparation.) Strain, then funnel into a pump-dispenser container.

Nine Easy-to-Find Soap Substitutes from Mother Nature

Makeup-remover pads (homemade or purchased at a cosmetic counter) premoistened with a freshener or astringent, can be used in an emergency or for midday oily-skin cleansing. Cold cream or cleansing cream (originating from a second-century Greek formula of olive oil, beeswax, and water which produces a cooling effect as the water evaporates) is fine for makeup removal but leaves a residue. In addition to the commercial foaming-liquid facial cleansers that appear to have resulted from a mating between cleansing cream and shampoo, Mother Nature offers soap equivalents. Indians in Columbia and in the Southwest of North America created an acceptable cleanser from chopped yucca roots. Botanicals such as soapbark, soapberry, soapwort, and the flowers of the sweet pepper bush were used by American Indians and early pioneers. The following cleansers are more convenient:

- **Alcohol,** mixed with water, was the cleansing solution recommended to travelers in the nineteenth century. (They were also advised to wash as infrequently as possible.)

- **Ammonia,** in the proportions of 1/4 teaspoon ammonia to 1 quart of water, is said to clean out the pores and take the place of soap. (Warning: don't use near your eyes.)

- **Glycerin,** smoothed on and wiped off, is believed to thoroughly cleanse your face.

- **Kelp granules,** blended with white vegetable shortening in the proportions of 1 teaspoon kelp to 2 tablespoons shortening, have healing as well as cleansing properties. Work the mixture into your face with a soft, moist sponge; remove with a damp washcloth.

- **Milk** is amazingly versatile. Plain whole milk, applied with a cotton ball and tissued off, replaces soap and water for a dry-skin cleanser. For normal or oily skin: make a paste with instant, nonfat dry milk and water, gently massage your face with the mixture, then rinse off with lukewarm water.

  Sour cream is an enriching cleanser for dry skin. To increase its benefits, squeeze the contents of a 5,000-IU vitamin A capsule into 1/2 cup of sour cream. Blend thoroughly and store in the refrigerator.

  Yogurt, with or without the addition of a capsuleful of vitamin A in each half cup, can replace soap for normal or combination skin.

- **Oatmeal** can be ground to a powder or used as-is. Dry oatmeal mixed to a paste with milk or cream, then smoothed on and rinsed off, is an exemplary soap substitute.

- **Oil** was the cleanser for the glamour-conscious Golden-Age Greeks, who did not use soap. They oiled their faces and bodies, scraped off the excess, and left a thin film to conserve their skin's moisture. You can follow their precept by smoothing on any vegetable or nut oil and wiping it off with a tissue.

- **Potato** (raw), grated and massaged into your face, then removed with a wet washcloth, is an effective cleanser with blemish-healing properties.

- **Wheat flour,** mixed to a paste with a little water, cleanses and smoothes skin when massaged in and rinsed off.

Ten Deep-Cleaning Exfoliants That Clean and Protect Your Skin Without Harsh Chemicals or Irritants

The dead cells clinging to your skin are oldies, not goodies. If they aren't sloughed off occasionally, they can enlarge your pores, muddy your complexion, and prevent their replacements from emerging. Shaving deposes most of this debris for men. Barbers recommend that electric-shaver users lather up and shave with a blade razor once a week. Dermatologists suggest occasional deep cleaning of facial areas that aren't de-whiskered.

The sloughing process (exfoliating or epidermabrading) should not be irritating. "Scrub" is a misnomer in that you don't "scrub"; you smooth, pat, or gently massage the exfoliant onto your clean, moist face, then rinse it off, pat dry, and apply your toner and moisturizer. How frequently you need to deep clean depends on your skin: from every day (if it looks dull, is very oily, or feels rough), to once a month if it is clear, dry, and sensitive. "Combination skin" may rate a weekly epidermabrasion on only the forehead, nose, and chin. Summer's upbeat schedule of increased cell production and shedding may call for more frequent sloughing. A complexion brush, moistened and stroked with feathery, rotary motions from throat to forehead over your usual cleanser may suffice; any of the following deep-cleaning exfoliants will also speed the departure of unwanted dead skin cells.

Almond meal

Almond meal smoothes skin while it cleanses. Make a thin paste with a tablespoon of almond meal and water, milk, and/or honey.

Almond-citrus oatmeal sounds like a breakfast cereal but is intended for external feeding: Mix 1/4 cup of leftover, cooked oatmeal with 1/4 cup almond meal and 1 teaspoon *each* dried lemon and orange peel. Store in a wide-mouth jar. To use: scoop a spoonful of the mixture into the palm of your hand, drizzle in a bit of hot water, then massage your face with gentle, circular motions. Rinse off with tepid water.

Almond-lanolin-egg is excellent for dry skins. You can make enough for several scrubs by combining the following ingredients in an electric blender and refrigerating the mixture.

1/3 cup almond meal

1/4 cup lanolin

1 raw egg yolk

1 teaspoon *each* almond extract and honey

1/2 teaspoon tincture of benzoin

Almond-papaya oil is another gently effective exfoliant that will keep for a week or two in the refrigerator.

1/3 cup mashed papaya (fresh or canned)

1/4 cup almond oil

2 tablespoons water-dispersible lecithin powder

2 teaspoons almond meal

1 teaspoon lemon extract

Whir in an electric blender until very smooth. Massage into the skin, gently remove with tissues; reapply and tissue off again, then rinse with tepid water.

Almond shortening is recommended for dry skins. Mix 1/4 cup *each* almond meal and white vegetable shortening with 2 teaspoons of honey. Store in a wide-mouth jar.

Almond yogurt, 1/4 cup yogurt blended with 1 tablespoon almond meal, is great for blemished skin.

Baking soda

Baking soda, mixed to a thin paste with water and smoothed over the face, is an anti-inflammatory agent as well as an exfoliant. Do not scrub with the soda, simply rinse it off with splashes of water.

Cornmeal

Cornmeal deep cleans and softens. Wet your face with warm water, moisten a tablespoon of yellow cornmeal with water or milk, then rub it gently into your skin with fingers or a complexion brush. Remove with a washcloth, rinse with cool water. (Note: Preparing the cornmeal paste in advance reduces its coarseness.)

Cornmeal-verbena cleanser can be made by softening 1/2 teaspoon of dried lemon verbena in 1 tablespoon warm water for 2 minutes, then stirring in 2 tablespoons cornmeal, plus additional water if needed, to make a thick paste.

Lemon or lime

Lemon face peel is good for normal or oily skin. Combine the grated rind and juice from one lemon. Cover and let stand for 8 hours. Pat the mixture over your face, let dry, then remove by gently rubbing with a damp washcloth. Rinse with cool water and apply a moisturizer.

- **Lemon scrubber.** Juice a lemon half (reserve the juice for other use), scoop out the lemon pulp and mix it with 2 tablespoons yogurt plus enough almond meal, cornmeal, or oatmeal to make a thick paste. Press the mixture into the lemon shell and wrap it in moistened cheesecloth. Rub the open end of the scrubber over your face for several minutes. Remove its traces, along with expired skin cells, with a damp cloth.

- **Lime juice,** diluted in the proportions of 1/2 lime to 1 cup warm water, can be used to dissolve the flaky top layer of skin. Dip a washcloth in the liquid, squeeze out the excess and cover your face for several minutes, then gently rub with the washcloth before rinsing off.

Milk

Milk can be used for a before-bed exfoliant-soother. Mix 2 tablespoons powdered whole milk with enough water to make a thick paste. Spread over your face and throat, rub in with fingers or a complexion brush, rinse off with tepid water. Apply a second coating of the milk paste and let it dry for a minute or so until it is sufficiently rubbery to roll off with your fingers. After rolling off this puttylike film, do not rinse and do not put anything else on your skin; the milk residue will continue conditioning your skin overnight.

Oatmeal

Oatmeal is a superb cleaner-softener. You can tie a handful of dry oatmeal in a square of gauze, swish it around in warm water, rub it over your freshly cleansed face, then let the oatmeal liquid dry for about 5 minutes before rinsing off.

Or, you can make a paste from oatmeal and water, milk, cream, or yogurt; smooth it over your face and throat, and let it dry before rinsing off. Caution: Oatmeal paste can be messy to apply, and hazardous to your skin if you live with a cat. One feline fancier spread a beach towel on the floor to protect it from oatmeal droplets, then lay down on the towel while the mixture dried on her face. She smiled as her affectionate tabby licked off some of the oatmeal paste. She was shocked upright when the cat took a bite that included part of her chin!

Papaya tea

Papaya tea contains an enzyme that dissolves surface cell debris. Squeeze a washcloth in strong, hot, papaya (or papaya-mint) tea. Cover your face with the cloth for a total of 15 minutes, redipping and rewringing every 2 or 3 minutes. Or, immerse a papaya tea bag in enough boiling water to cover it, let cool until comfortably warm, then smooth the tea bag over your face. Allow the liquid to dry before rinsing off.

Pineapple

The bromelain enzyme in fresh pineapple is another dead-cell dissolver. Press the juice out of a slice of fresh pineapple or puree fresh pineapple chunks in a blender. Smooth over your face and let dry. Rub gently with a dry washcloth before removing with a wet washcloth. To intensify the exfoliating benefits, saturate strips of gauze or cotton cloth with the pineapple juice and apply as a 5-minute compress over your original coating.

Pineapple-carrot juice is advised for blemished skin. Mix equal amounts of fresh pineapple juice and carrot juice and use as directed above.

Salt: epsom, sea, and table

Blend 1/2 teaspoon *each* epsom salt, and table salt (or 1 teaspoon sea salt) with 1 tablespoon white vegetable shortening. Massage into your skin with your fingertips for 3 minutes. Leave on your face if you are going to "steam" as part of a facial (see Chapter 5), or remove with warm water and a washcloth.

Instead of epidermabrasion, you can indulge in a "salabrasion" every week or two by dissolving 1 teaspoon *each* epsom salt and table salt (or 2 teaspoons sea salt) in 1/4 cup hot water, sponging on the saline solution, and allowing it to dry before rinsing off with warm water.

Buttermilk salt is recommended for oily skin. Mix a spoonful of buttermilk with enough table salt to make a grainy scrub. Massage into your face, then rinse off.

Sunflower scrub

Sunflower scrub, made by mixing ground sunflower seeds with milk, can be massaged in and rinsed off; or the ground seeds may be substituted for almond meal in any exfoliant.

Back to Basics: The *Right* Way to Wash Your Face

Step-by-step directions for this fundamental process seem as ridiculous as instruction for tying shoe laces, but every skin care expert has a long list of adamant rules. Water—hot versus warm, cold versus cool—is a prime bone of contention. Rinsing with a washcloth or splashing with water a certain number of times is another point of debate, "Wash with hot, rinse with cold" proponents contend this method cleanses more efficiently, opens and closes pores, and stimulates circulation. Other dermatologists declare that hot rinsing arouses the *lipids* (oil glands) into reestablishing the skin's pH balance. The "warm/cool" and the "keep it tepid" brigade believe that skin should never be shocked with either hot or cold, and agree with the American Medical Association's statement that pores neither open nor close.[149] Among these extremes are some facts: skin around the pores does contract and expand to have the effect of opening and closing pores; warm-to-hot water is comfortable for washing; and a splash of cold water is refreshing as a final rinse. Here's the basic process for properly washing your face:

1. Moisten your face with water. Work up a lather by rubbing the soap between wet palms. Using your fingertips (not the bar of soap), massage the lather into your face and throat.

2. Rinse thoroughly with a washcloth or with splashes of water. A three-to-one ratio of rinsing time to lathering time is considered adequate; the important thing is that you remove all of the soap so any caustic it contains won't burn your face, and so your face won't be left with the film equivalent of a bathtub ring.

3. Blot dry with a soft towel; vigorous rubbing with coarse material aggravates and tugs at your skin.

❧ 3 ❧

Toning: Fresheners & Astringents Tailor-made to Fit Your Face

Thorough cleansing removes more than makeup, grime, and cellular debris: it strips your skin of its protective shield. Toners, fresheners and astringents restore the pH balance of the acid mantle; remove any lingering vestiges of makeup, oily cleanser, or soap film; make pores seem smaller and fine wrinkles less noticeable. They should not be harsh enough to irritate your skin. If your face is sensitive and powdery-dry, rose water or other botanical water may be all you need; if it is extremely oily, a stronger astringent will dispense with the excess sebum as it tones.

How to Make Your Own Skin-Care Products

According to Federal Regulations Code #21, cosmetics are "articles to be applied to the body for cleaning, beautifying, promoting attractiveness or altering the appearance," and are not subject to the same standards as foods and drugs. We may feel condescendingly superior to the sixteenth-century courtesans who wasted away as a result of powdering their faces with white lead, but label-scrutinizing can reveal some surprises about the cosmetics now on the market. The same chemicals used in insecticides are often incorporated in beauty products to prolong shelf life,[161] formaldehyde may be included in lotions as well as in nail hard-

21

eners,[12] while other potentially hazardous ingredients contribute color and scent to beautify the product, not the skin to which they are applied. It's no longer "un-macho" for men to care for their skin; industry analysts reveal that sales of masculine cosmetic preparations rose from 20 million in 1985 to 40 million in 1987. Skin bracers and after shave lotions—consisting primarily of alcohol, water and scent—provide little more than sting.

Concocting your own natural cosmetics is amazingly easy and rewarding. You can tailor the formulas to fit your face. If your skin is a

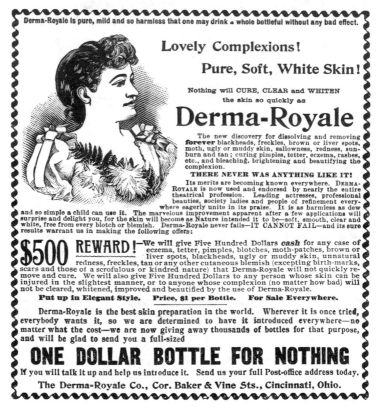

This 1890's beauty product may not have been as miraculous as advertised, but it was safe to drink.

normal combination, you can bottle two-thirds of your prepared toner-astringent to use on your oily T-zone; then dilute the remainder for toning your cheeks and throat. By pouring a little of the full-strength mixture over pressed-cotton puffs in an airtight container, you can manufacture your own makeup-remover/skin-freshener pads.

EQUIPMENT AND INGREDIENTS: Your "cosmetics lab" requires only standard measuring spoons and cups, an enamel or glass pan, a fine sieve, and a funnel. A medicine cup or jigger with graduated markings is a convenient time saver (one fluid ounce equals two tablespoons): if your tap water contains chlorine or fluoride, you may have more satisfactory results if you use bottled water. For aesthetic appeal, you can add a few drops of vegetable food coloring, or exotic scents from the essential oils, fragrant oils, or extracts available in beauty supply houses, health food stores, or supermarkets. Alcohol, benzoin, vinegar, and witch hazel are natural preservatives for your lotions and potions. Fruits and vegetables are perishable, however, so it is wise to prepare small quantities and refrigerate any surplus.

How to Coddle Your Complexion—and Budget—with Eight Skin-firming Mixtures

Aromatic, botanical waters

These waters may be used alone for a mild toner or added to astringents as a "strength reducer." For increased astringency, stir in one or two teaspoons of lemon juice. For skin texturizing and product preserving, add a tablespoon of tincture of benzoin. As a bonus, you can mix a bit of lemon juice with the strained botanical remains and utilize them as a facial pack.

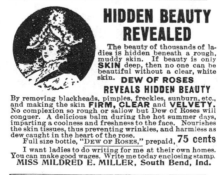

- **Rose water**, the most versatile beauty liquid, can be purchased in pharmacies. If you would rather do it yourself, you can acquire *rose otto* (attar of roses, rose oil) by having a lackey collect the oil floating on your moatful of drifting rose petals—as did a sixteenth-century Persian princess—follow the example set by

Napolean's Josephine who considered rose water a love potion and cultivated over 250 different types of roses, or opt for one of these methods:

Attar of roses: Fill a large jar with unsprayed, freshly picked, rose petals. Add distilled water to cover, then top with a fine screen. Place the jar in the sunshine each day, bring it indoors at night. As the rose oil rises to the surface, lift it off with cotton balls and squeeze it into a small glass vial with a tight lid. Continue the process for a week or until no more oil appears.

Rose water from attar of roses: Dissolve 1/4 teaspoon of the rose oil in 1/2 cup rubbing alcohol. Add 5 cups distilled water, mix thoroughly, then decant into small bottles for storage.

Rose water astringent: Mix 3/4 cup rose water with 1/4 cup rubbing alcohol—adjust to the desired degree of tingle by adding more of either liquid.

Quicker, easier and milder *rose water* can be produced by following the directions given with floral waters, below.

- **Floral waters.** Acacia flowers, clover blooms, elderflowers, orange or lemon blossoms and leaves, rose petals or buds, or violets can be simmered in just enough water to cover, allowed to cool, then strained, and the liquid bottled.

- **Herbal waters** have long been used by men as well as women to firm skin tissue and retain its youthfulness. To make camomile, chervil, comfrey or sage water: Place 3/4 cup of the fresh herb in a glass jar with 1 cup of water. Cover tightly and shake each morning and evening for 2 weeks. Strain and bottle.

    A quick mint tonic can be made by liquefying a handful of fresh mint leaves with an ice cube in an electric blender.

- **Vegetable waters.** Stir 1/2 cup grated cucumber, or 1/2 cup finely minced celery and leaves, with 1 cup of water. Let stand for 1 hour, then strain through doubled cheesecloth and squeeze out all the liquid. Bottle and refrigerate.

    Cucumber or celery astringent can be made to order by mixing 1/4 cup of the vegetable water with a tablespoon or so of rubbing alcohol, vodka, or witch hazel.

Refreshing tea toners

Herbal teas, made double-strength and steeped for several hours, are not only facial toners with mildly astringent properties; they provide a facial treatment if allowed to dry on your skin for 30 minutes. Comfrey or camomile tea offers the same skin firming benefits as a "water" made from the fresh herb. Chervil tea is ideal for fair skin. Mint or sage tea is a gentle astringent for normal, combination, or oily skin.

- *Camomile-rosemary refresher*, made from 2 camomile tea bags plus 1 tablespoon dried rosemary steeped in 1-1/2 cups water and strained, is especially recommended as a postexercise unisex skin refresher.

- *Strawberry-mint tea*, prepared by steeping 1 tea bag of each in 1 cup of boiling water, is a delightfully scented skin freshener-toner.

Cosmetic vinegars

Apple cider vinegar, white vinegar, or wine vinegar can be splashed on as an acid-mantle restorer when mixed with water in the proportions of one teaspoon to one tablespoon of vinegar to each half-cup of water, depending on personal preference and the dryness of your skin. Cosmetic vinegars, first concocted by medieval alchemists and still sold in European herb shops, have olfactory appeal as well as additional benefits, and are used as after-shave lotions by German barbers. When you make your own, dilute with a little rose water or other botanical water for use as a toner on oily skin and dilute with a lot of the water for dry-skin toning.

- *Floral vinegars*. Pour 2 cups slightly warmed white vinegar over 2 cups fresh, unsprayed petals from carnations, honeysuckle, lavender, roses, violets, or other scented flowers. Mix well. Steep in a lidded glass container for 2 weeks, shaking daily, then strain the liquid into a smaller glass bottle.

- *Herbal vinegars*. Prepare from camomile, dill, lemon grass, rosemary, sweet basil, thyme, or other pungent herb by pouring 2 cups of warm white vinegar over 1 cup of fresh snippets (or 1/4 cup of the dried herb), and following the directions for floral vinegars.

  Instant mint vinegar. Mix 1 cup cider vinegar, 1 cup boiling water, and 1/4 teaspoon oil of peppermint. For scent, add 1/4 teaspoon oil of rose geranium.

  Minute mint vinegar. Mix 1 cup double-strength peppermint tea with 1 cup cider vinegar.

  Rose-camomile vinegar. Steep 1 cup fresh rose petals and 1/2 cup fresh (or 2 tablespoons dried) camomile flowers in 2 cups white wine vinegar for 1 week. Strain, then add 1 cup rose water to the liquid.

Scented vinegar. Steep 1 tablespoon *each* dried lavender, mint, rosemary, and thyme in 1 quart white vinegar for 2 weeks, shaking the bottle daily. Strain and bottle.

Variegated vinegar. Pour 1 pint of boiling white vinegar over 1/4 cup *each* fresh camomile, orange flowers, orange leaves, orange peel, rosebuds, rose hips, rose leaves, and white willow bark. (The willow bark may be omitted, and 2 teaspoons dried camomile substituted for fresh, if desired.) Let the mixture steep in a tightly closed container, shaking the bottle once each day, until the botanicals lose their color. Strain, add 1 cup rose water, let settle for a few days, then decant the clear liquid into a smaller bottle.

- *Lemon vinegar.* For a mild astringent that requires no advance preparation or refrigerated storage: Blend 1/2 cup water with 1/4 cup apple cider vinegar and 1 teaspoon lemon extract. Shake well before using.

- *Strawberry vinegar:* Stir 1/4 cup mashed ripe strawberries into 1/2 cup white vinegar. Cover and let stand for several hours, then strain out the seeds and blend the liquid with 1/4 cup rose water.

Peroxide

Hydrogen peroxide, in the 3 percent solution available from drug stores, is a gentle toner and an antiseptic that helps eradicate existing blemishes and prevent new ones from appearing. (When used daily, it also bleaches facial hair—be cautious around your eyebrows and hairline.) Peroxide gradually loses strength and eventually turns into just plain water—discard it after the expiration date printed on the bottle.

Witch hazel

The commercial product is a freshening-toning-antiseptic liquid extracted with alcohol from the leaves or bark of the witch hazel shrub, then reduced with water. For a quick-mix freshener or after-shave with sparkle: combine 1/4 cup witch hazel with 1 teaspoon lemon or peppermint extract from the kitchen shelf.

If your skin is especially dry dilute the witch hazel with rose water, or make your own alcohol-free witch hazel water by boiling 3 tablespoons witch hazel leaves or bark in 2 cups of water for 5 minutes. Let cool, then strain and bottle.

Cosmetic cocktails

Your face needn't be a teetotaler, even if you are. Vodka has less odor than rubbing alcohol and is a smoother mixer for toners and astringents.

- *Russian rose refresher*. Pour 1/2 cup rose water into a glass or plastic bottle with a screw cap. Add 1/4 cup 80-proof vodka and 1/4 teaspoon glycerin. Shake to blend. Test on your skin, then adjust for the precise amount of tingle you want by adding either vodka or rose water.

Paul and Jennifer had a shelf cluttered with skin bracers and fresheners, each of which was either too harsh or too mild. Weary of playing Goldilocks sampling the bears' porridge, Jennifer concocted her own "just right" Russian refresher and was so delighted with the results she decided to create a lotion for Paul.

Holiday After-Shave

1/4 cup white rum

2 tablespoons double-strength camomile tea

1/4 teaspoon rum extract

2 drops maple flavoring

Paul says it smells like a Christmas party and reminds him of their vacation breakfasts in Vermont. He is so happy to have his "just right, just for him" lotion that Jennifer hasn't admitted she was thinking of the aroma of her father's pipe tobacco when she added the rum and maple flavorings!

- *Whiskey toner*. Blend 1/3 cup whiskey with 1 teaspoon tincture of benzoin. Add 1 cup water, stopper tightly, then shake. This was a favorite, "perfectly harmless," complexion reviver during the 1800s. The instructions called for diluting the mixture with more water, if desired, sponging it over the face and throat, and letting it dry.

Fruitful fresheners

- *Apple juice* gives your face a refreshing lift.
- *Grape*. Split a grape, remove any seeds, then run the cut halves over your face and throat for toning and refreshing.

- *Grapefruit juice.* Squeeze a teaspoonful of fresh grapefruit juice into the palm of your hand. Smooth over your face and throat.

- *Lemon,* because of its astringent properties, is especially recommended for oily skins.

    Cooked lemon astringent: Cook 1 chopped lemon with 1/2 cup water in a small, covered pan until tender. Whir in an electric blender, strain to remove any fragments of peel, then dilute with water to the desired strength.

    Lemon frost: To duplicate a famous salon's skin refresher used as an after-shave or after-masque toner: Blender whir 1/4 cup *each* distilled water and lemon juice with 2 ice cubes and 1 teaspoon olive oil.

    Lemon milk: Stir 1 tablespoon lemon juice into 1/4 cup milk. Apply generously, then blot off the excess. For a stronger solution, substitute water for milk.

    Lemon-lime freshener: In an 8-ounce bottle, combine 1/3 cup water, 1 tablespoon *each* lemon juice and lime juice, and 1/2 teaspoon tincture of benzoin. Stopper tightly, shake to blend, then refrigerate until ready to use.

- *Orange or tangerine* slices or segments may be smoothed over the face and throat for freshening and toning.

Vegetable tonics

- *Celery astringent:* Finely chop 1 large rib of celery with leaves. Simmer, covered, in 1 cup water for 20 minutes. Strain, stir in 1/4 cup rubbing alcohol and 2 teaspoons tincture of benzoin.

- *Cucumber* is a centuries-old complexion aid still used in exclusive beauty salons and included in some of the more expensive commercial cosmetics. You can acquire cucumber's mildly astringent benefits by rubbing the meaty side of a strip of its peeling, or a slice of raw cucumber, over your face.

    Cucumber-citrus astringent: Pour the juice from half a lemon and half an orange into the container of an electric blender. Add half a cucumber, cut in chunks, and whir on high speed for a few seconds. Strain, then stir in a tablespoon of rubbing alcohol, vodka, or witch hazel.

    Cucumber-lettuce lotion is a no-alcohol astringent with masculine as well as feminine appeal. Boil the dark, outer leaves of a head of leaf lettuce in 1 cup water. Let stand until cool. Strain, then combine the liquid with the strained juice from a cucumber liquefied in an electric blender.

Cucumber milk is a mild toner for after cleansing (or after shaving) or for mutual midday skin refreshing. Liquefy enough chopped cucumber to produce 1/4 cup strained juice, then add 2 tablespoons milk.

Cucumber-witch hazel is recommended for normal or oily skin. Liquefy half a cucumber (chopped) with 2 tablespoons water and 1 teaspoon honey in an electric blender. Strain, discard the pulp, then add enough witch hazel to make 1 cup. Chill before using. For very oily skin: Mix 1/4 cup of liquefied, strained cucumber juice with an equal amount of commercial witch hazel.

Cooked cucumber freshener: Cut half a cucumber in chunks and whir in a blender with 1/2 cup water. (Or, mince the cucumber and stir into 1/2 cup water.) Simmer in a covered saucepan for 20 minutes and let stand to cool. Strain through doubled cheesecloth, squeeze the liquid into a small bowl, then stir in tincture of benzoin, a few drops at a time, until the cucumber takes on a milky appearance.

- *Potato*. For an instant freshener-toner, rub a slice of raw potato over your face and throat.

- *Tomato*, sliced and rubbed over your skin (or mashed, smeared on and wiped off) is a mildly astringent toner.

Five Custom-Made Complexion Toners, Tonics, and Astringents

Here are five complexion refreshers you can make at home:

1. *Almond flower milk*. For a tissue building skin refresher, whir 1/4 cup almond meal in an electric blender with enough rose water to form a loosely flowing lotion. Strain, stir in 1/4 teaspoon tincture of benzoin, then decant into an attractive container.

2. *Benzoin water*. The May 1895 issue of *The Delineator* states that the most efficacious spring tonic for enervated skin is a drop of benzoin beaten into 1/4 cup water. It is to be sponged over a thoroughly clean face and throat, then allowed to dry without rinsing. For a skin-firming toner: mix 1/4 teaspoon tincture of benzoin with 1/4 cup rose water and apply with a cotton ball. Do not rinse off.

3. *Glycerin*, mixed with rose water or other aromatic water, is an old-fashioned toner for dry to normal complexions. Test with the

proportions of 1/4 teaspoon glycerin to 1/2 cup of the water, then add more glycerin if desired.

4. *Herbal astringent* for oily skin: Steep 1 tea bag *each* camomile and peppermint in 1 cup boiling water until cool. Remove the tea bags (pressing out all the liquid) and stir in 3 tablespoons witch hazel, 1 teaspoon vinegar, and 1 teaspoon tincture of benzoin. If your skin is encumbered by blemishes, you can add the antiseptic qualities of boric acid by stirring in 1/4 teaspoon of crystalline powder.

5. *Honey* can be shaken with mineral water or any botanical water to make a nonsticky, skin-smoothing toner. One tablespoon honey to 1/2 cup of the water is the usual ratio.

How Ice and Snow Can Tighten Pores and Refine Your Skin

Modern dermatologists warn against shocking the skin with temperature extremes, and cite laboratory tests showing that tiny capillaries near the surface can become so traumatized that they will mar your appearance with spidery red veins. Nevertheless, beauty conscious women have been employing ice or snow for skin-refining and pore-tightening for hundreds of years. As one 93-year-old charmer replied when asked for the secret of her clear, fine-textured complexion, "I don't have any secret. All I've ever done is what my mother did: smooth on a touch of olive oil at night, and wash with soap and water—rinse thoroughly, then rub an ice cube over my face. Of course," she admitted with a smile, "when I was young, we went out and scooped up a handful of snow in the wintertime, or chipped a piece off a block of ice in the summer—we didn't have ice cubes." Our refrigerator-freezers offer more interesting alternatives.

- *Ice diving*: Fill the bathroom sink with cold water and two trays of ice cubes. Pin your hair back, or don a shower cap. Dip your face in the icy water for as long as you can hold your breath. Blot almost dry, then apply your moisturizer. A famous actor credits his daily ice dive (without the shower cap) for his non-receding hairline as well as his youthful-appearing skin.

- *Lemon freeze*: Combine strained fresh lemon juice and water to the degree of astringency you prefer. Partially fill an ice cube tray (your frozen cubes need not to be more than one-half an inch thick), freeze, pop out, and store in a plastic bag in the freezer. To use: Lightly rub one of the icy rectangles over your face. Tissue off the excess lemon liquid, along with any surplus skin oil.

- *Super ice*: This duplicates the effects of "cold iron" salon treatments to increase circulation, wake up a weary face, and leave your complexion firm and dewy fresh.

Mix 1/2 cup bottled mineral water with 1/2 cup of your favorite freshener and 1/4 teaspoon alum. Pour into an ice cube tray, freeze, pop out, and store in an airtight container in the freezer. When you rub a cube over your face, pause a few seconds over any noticeable lines or wrinkles before blotting off the excess liquid.

❧ 4 ❧

Moisturizers & Night Nourishers for Softer, More Supple Skin

Who needs to moisturize? Almost everyone. *Cleansing* strips away the protective acid mantle and surface oil; *toning* restores the pH balance so the sebaceous glands (which commence their withering-away decline when we reach the age of 25) can proceed with their skin-lubricating chores; *moisturizing* helps retain the radiantly unwrinkled bloom of youth by sealing in water and replenishing some of the precious oils reduced by aging or removed during cleansing and toning. Race, gender, and inherited tendencies are largely responsible for allover dry or always-oily skin; normal skin is a mosaic combination of slightly dry and slightly oily. Caucasian women have drier skin than women of black, Latin, or oriental origin. Men of all nationalities have more productive sebaceous glands than their female counterparts and may be able to wait until they are in their forties before moisturizing dry areas. We can't alter our ancestry or our genes, but we can make the most of the skin we have by moisturizing when and where required.

Water: Nature's Secret for Dewy-fresh Skin

Water (comprising 70 to 90 percent of skin, other body tissues, and blood) is Mother Nature's secret for dewy-fresh skin. As skin physiologist Dr. Peter T. Puglise explains in the January 1988 issue of *Health*, water moves through the body to the surface in a process called "transepidermal water loss," leaving skin pleasingly plump and firm. If your system is deficient in water, the skin's upper layers become dry and brittle. Drinking at least six glasses of water daily and eating fluid-rich fruits and vegetables helps normalize dry or oily conditions, and is essential for preventing your body from hoarding its necessary moisture at the expense of your skin. In addition to internal liquid refreshment, skin requires external water replenishing. Supplying this water from the outside is something of a paradox: extended immersion first bloats and puffs your skin, then leaves it looking like a shriveled prune; water applied and allowed to evaporate untended carries away some of the skin's own moisture. Moderation in watery contacts, plus *humecants*, *emollients*, and *occlusives* (see Glossary) smoothed over slightly damp skin, resolve the dilemma.

Tips on Moisturizing Your Skin

Dry skin

Facial skin reveals crinkly-wrinkly signs sooner than body skin because of exposure to the elements and more frequent cleansings. Sales of masculine moisturizers are mounting as men, too, strive to prevent the telltale evidence of aging, and wrinkle-prone dry skin is the most common problem besetting over-30 women. Including two tablespoons of unsaturated oil in your diet and taking a Vitamin A supplement may lessen dry-skin discomfort and flakiness. Contrary to advertisements generated by cosmetic promoters, however, slathering on globs of elegantly packaged skin rejuvenators won't slow Father Time. Neither collagen nor elastin can be assimilated from topical application, and, according to Dr. Erno Lazlo and other skin care experts,[45, 83] smothering your skin with heavy creams may enlarge pores, cause facial blemishes, and weaken its elasticity to such an extent that it will droop and sag with nature's gravitational pull. Moistening with water, then applying a thin film of air-excluding moisturizer, restores its suppleness.[149]

NIGHT MOISTURIZING: Complete your cleansing-toning routine with a splash of water or a water-misting. Pat almost dry with a soft towel, then smooth moisturizer from bosom to hairline. For the ultimate benefit, allow five minutes for immediate absorption (cover your face and throat with warm washcloths to hasten penetration) then blot off any excess moisturizer with a tissue. Men may elect to skip the toner but should moisturize the delicate skin around the eye area which contains few oil glands.

DAY MOISTURIZING: Even if you use a makeup foundation that includes a moisturizer, caressing a touch of your natural moisturizer over the freshly cleansed, toned, and dampened skin on your throat, cheeks, and around your eyes can pay beautiful dividends. Men are advised to follow a "double-dose" routine of applying moisturizer immediately after shaving, waiting ten minutes, then moisturizing again.

Oily skin

Oiliness, like dryness, varies with time, temperature, your endocrine system, and your emotions (stress may be responsible for a sudden outburst of oily-skin problems[163]). Cutting back on fried foods, pastries, and other saturated food fats may reduce the amount of excess oil accumulating on your epidermis. If your skin is extremely oily, three or four daily cleansings may be in order and little or no moisturizing necessary before you reach the 30-year milepost. After that point, the skin around your eyes and mouth and on your throat may benefit from a nightly moisturizing, plus a mere touch of moisturizer in the morning. If your oily skin is scaly, using a deep-cleaning exfoliant on alternate nights, and following the treatment with a light coating of moisturizer often corrects the problem.

Combination skin

For most of us, oily areas are concentrated in the T-zone of forehead, nose, chin, with drier, moisture-thirsty skin covering the rest of the face and throat. If twice-daily allover moisturizing accentuates the oiliness, experiment with "spot moisturizing" on alternate nights and for daytime care.

When to Remoisturize

Here are three general guidelines on when to remoisturize your skin:

1. Before and after your face is exposed to wind or extremely hot or cold outdoor temperatures, or when it has had an encounter with ocean spray, swimming-pool water, or falling snow or rain.

2. When you're sitting near an open fire, when your culinary endeavors require a lot of oven-door opening and closing, or when you use hot rollers, a curling iron, or a hair dryer on its high setting.

3. When the relative humidity is low, as in pressurized airplanes, overheated rooms, and desert climates. Under these conditions your body contains a higher percentage of fluid than the air around it and loses water rapidly.

Do-It-Yourself Moisturizers That Cost Little and Replenish Much

Ancient Greeks anointed themselves with sweet oil, American Indians and hardy pioneers smeared on bear grease or skunk oil; we have many other options. To increase the benefits from your moisturizer you can incorporate vitamins A and E by snipping capsules and squeezing the contents into your homemade cosmetic. Comfrey is another beneficial additive; *allantoin*, comfrey's major component, promotes tissue building, cell restoring, and healing. Some cosmetic manufacturers blend comfrey into their night creams; you can mix a spoonful of comfrey tea with your own moisturizer, or reap even more of allantoin's skin-strengthening rewards by applying cooled comfrey tea instead of water before smoothing on your night nourisher.

Cocoa butter, oils, and petroleum jelly

These ready-to-use moisturizers double as a base for makeup and are ideal for both men and women.

- *For dry skin*: cocoa butter; almond, castor, olive, peanut, and wheat germ oils.

- *For oily skin*: corn, cottonseed, poppyseed, safflower, sesame, and sunflower seed oils.

- *For normal skin*: any of the above (warmed peanut oil is said to work wonders when massaged into a "scrawny" neck[74]) or avocado, coconut, mink, or soy oils.

Lanolin and mineral oil are effective occlusives but lanolin may instigate skin problems for those allergic to wool; mineral oil sometimes leaves an irritating residue and is suspected of robbing the body of fat-soluble vitamins. If you can wear wool comfortably, you can make a nurturing moisturizer by warming 1/4 cup lanolin in the top of a double boiler, stirring in 1/4 cup safflower oil, then adding 5,000 IU vitamin A and 100 IU vitamin E from pierced capsules.

This femme fatale formula is a wonder-working oil mixture similar to the one Cleopatra's handmaidens lavishly applied and then scooped off with a spatula-like "strygil."

3 tablespoons *each* safflower and sesame oil

2 tablespoons *each* avocado and peanut oil

1 tablespoon *each* olive oil and wheat germ oil

5 drops of perfume oil (optional)—musk, rose, geranium, or other favorite

Petroleum jelly does not provide the nourishment of natural oils, yet is effective, innocuous, and versatile. Cathy discovered it to be an indispensable traveling companion when car trouble turned an afternoon drive into a weekend adventure. The mountain lodge offered comfortable accommodations and a magnificent dining room. Behind racks of candy and potato chips in the service-station office, Jason found toothbrushes and a disposable razor, but the only beauty product available was a jar of petroleum jelly. Cathy used it to remove her makeup and as a night cream. They both utilized it as hand lotion, smoothed it on their chapped lips and over their arms and faces when they went exploring in the high altitude sunlight—and had enough left to polish their dusty shoes before going to dinner!

Fruits

Lemon juice or orange juice blended with olive oil is a time-tested keep-it-supple skin moisturizer. Apples contain *malic acid*, a moisturizing agent. Peaches-and-cream complexions have been attributed to smoothing on a blender-whirred mixture of half a peeled peach or apple and a dollop of cream.

- *Peach moisturizer for dry or normal skin*: In an electric blender, whir 1 chopped, peeled peach with 1/4 cup almond oil, 3 tablespoons rose water, 4 drops tincture of benzoin, and (if desired) a few drops of orange oil or other perfume. Strain and store in the refrigerator.

- *Fruit cream for normal or oily skin*: Mash and squeeze through cheesecloth (or liquefy in a blender and strain) enough chopped fresh apricot, honeydew melon, peach, or strawberries to produce 2 tablespoons of juice. Heat 1/4 cup almond oil and 1/2 ounce white beeswax or paraffin in the top of a double boiler until the wax melts. Remove from the heat, beat in the fruit juice and 1/4 teaspoon tincture of benzoin. Continue beating until the mixture is fluffy, then transfer to a wide-mouth jar with a tightly fitting lid.

Glycerin

As described in an 1895 ladies' magazine, "Glycerine Emollient" is justly favored for pulling moisture into dry skin. The instructions call for bringing 1/2 cup glycerin to a boil, letting it cool, then adding 1/4 cup rose water.

Glycerin and honey, in the proportions of 3 tablespoons glycerin to 1 teaspoon honey, is recommended by modern skin-care experts as a wear-all-day or leave-on-all-night moisturizer.[93]

Lecithin

For a multipurpose moisturizer-makeup base-hand smoother, whir 1/2 cup almond *or* apricot kernel *or* avocado oil in an electric blender with 1/4 cup *each* water and water-dispersible lecithin powder. For more night-nourishing benefits, substitute 1/4 cup honey for the water.

Lecithin yogurt requires refrigeration and has a shorter life span, but it is a wonderful night cream you can whir up in the blender.

3 tablespoons water-dispersible lecithin powder

2 tablespoons *each* water and plain yogurt

2 tablespoons *each* avocado oil and wheat germ oil

2 teaspoons potato flour

5 drops of your favorite perfume (optional)

Mayonnaise

Mayonnaise (see Glossary for homemade recipe) can be massaged into a clean, damp face and throat whenever skin is dehydrated from exposure to sun, wind, or winter cold. With the excess blotted off after a few minutes' absorption time, mayonnaise is also a night cream.

Milk and cream

Sweet or sour milk or cream, buttermilk, or whey are all moisturizers especially recommended for irritated skin.

Miss Muffet's moisturizer: Add a lemon slice to 1/4 cup warm milk, cover and let stand for 2 hours. Strain and discard the curds which will have formed (or sit on your tuffet and eat them) then apply the liquid whey to your skin with a cotton ball.

Vegetables

For centuries, French women and men have moisturized their faces with lettuce juice; our rural ancestors used split fresh cucumbers to revive their dehydrated skins.

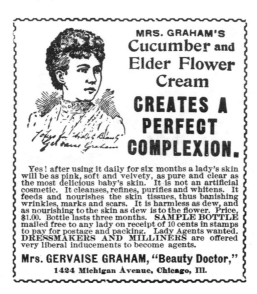

- *Cucumber cream*: Cut a 5/8-inch slice off one of the 2-1/2-inch-by-5-inch-by-5/8-inch cakes of paraffin sold for topping home-made jelly. Melt the half-ounce of paraffin in the top of a double boiler or in a a heat-proof glass bowl set in a pan of water over low heat. Stir in 1/4 cup almond oil a teaspoonful at a time. Puree a medium-size cucumber, chopped but not peeled, in an electric blender or food processor; strain through cheesecloth into the oil-paraffin mixture and blend thoroughly. Let the creamy mixture cool to room temperature, stirring several times to prevent crystals from forming, then transfer to a wide-mouth jar and store in the refrigerator for up to 2 months.

- *Montmartre Moisturizer*: Simmer lettuce leaves until tender in a lidded pan with just enough distilled water to cover. Let cool, strain off the liquid and apply as is, or blend a spoonful of it with an equal amount of yogurt. Refrigerate the surplus lettuce liquid.

Nighttime Nourishing:
Moisturizers That Work While You Sleep

In sixteenth-century Venice, beauty-conscious ladies slept with milk-soaked veal cutlets secured over their cheeks to moisturize and improve their complexions. We have more comfortable and less costly methods of nighttime nourishing. Besides those previously mentioned, a thin film of white vegetable shortening, soybean margarine, or milk blended with butter will seal in needed moisture. For more sophisticated skin nourishing, try one of these options.

Fruit and vegetable nourishers

- *Artichoke butter,* used nightly, helps tighten crinkled or "crepey" skin. To prepare a week's supply for refrigerator storage remove the heart from a cooked artichoke, mash it, then gradually work in 1/4 cup unsalted butter and 1/4 teaspoon tincture of benzoin.

- *Avocado.* Mash an avocado slice with a fork until it is the consistency of butter. Massage into your face and throat, let penetrate for 5 minutes, then tissue off the excess.

  Avocado cream. Melt 1 ounce white beeswax (or a 1-1/4-inch slice of paraffin) in the top of a double boiler, and add one fourth of an avocado (well mashed). Beat in 2 tablespoons apricot-kernel, almond or coconut oil plus 1 tablespoon lanolin if you are not allergic to wool. Add 2 tablespoons rose water and 1/4 teaspoon tincture of benzoin. Continue beating until the mixture solidifies, then refrigerate.

  Fruitless avocado cream. Melt 1 ounce white beeswax in the top of a double boiler. Beat in 1/4 cup avocado oil, 2 tablespoons rose water, 2 teaspoons lanolin, and 1/4 teaspoon tincture of benzoin. Beat until creamy.

- *Strawberries and tea* are a "dream treatment" for normal or combination skin. Mash a few ripe strawberries, squeeze through cheesecloth, then dilute with a spoonful of water and sponge over your face before going to bed. In the morning, rinse off the dried juice with warm chervil tea.

Gelatin-based night nourishers

These miraculous elixirs should be smoothed over clean, damp skin; allowed to penetrate for a few minutes, then blotted with a tissue. If you or your resident male are plagued by tiny under-the-skin bumps, add 1 teaspoon vitamin C crystals and a crushed aspirin to either of the following formulas and share the skin-leveling results. This may be just what the doctor would have ordered: salicylic acid (present in aspirin) is used for prescriptive skin treatments.

How to prepare the gelatin base: Measure out 1/2 cup water; place 2 tablespoons of the water in the container of an electric blender and sprinkle with 1-1/2 teaspoons unflavored gelatin. Allow the gelatin to soften while you bring the remainder of the water to a boil. Pour the boiling water into the blender and whir to dissolve the gelatin.

Nighttime formula for dry-normal-combination skin: To the gelatin base in the blender container, add:

1/2 cup almond oil (or avocado, olive, peanut, or wheat germ oil)

2 tablespoons water-dispersible lecithin powder or liquid lecithin

1 tablespoon castor oil

1 1/2 teaspoons cod liver oil

1 teaspoon dried, ground kelp

100 IU vitamin E (squeezed from a pierced capsule)

Blend on medium speed for 15 seconds, or until smooth. Refrigerate in a lightproof container.

- Variation for dry skin: Add 1 teaspoon glycerin and 1 teaspoon sesame oil before blending.
- Variation for combination skin with an oily T-zone: Add 2 tablespoons vodka before blending.
- Variation for skin with large pores, wrinkles and/or sags: Add 1 egg white, 1 teaspoon sesame oil, and 1 teaspoon vitamin C crystals before blending.

Nighttime formula for oily skin: To the gelatin base in the blender container, add:

1/2 cup sparkling mineral water

1 teaspoon glycerin

1 teaspoon dried, ground kelp

1/8 teaspoon vitamin C crystals

5000 IU "dry" vitamin A (from a 2-part capsule)

100 IU "dry" vitamin E (from a 2-part capsule)

Whir on medium speed for 15 seconds, or until smooth. Transfer to a lightproof container and refrigerate.

- Variation for oily skin with breakouts: Add 2 tablespoons vodka before blending.
- Variation for oily skin with enlarged pores: Increase the amount of vitamin C crystals to 1 teaspoon.
- Variation for oily skin with lines and sags: Increase the amount of vitamin C crystals to 1 teaspoon, and add 1/4 teaspoon alum before blending.

Oil creams

For a night cream that doubles as a body lotion, warm 3 tablespoons *each* corn oil and olive oil with 1 tablespoon almond oil in the top of a double boiler. Add 2 tablespoons distilled water and beat until creamy.

Wheat germ and honey moisturizer: It takes less than five minutes to whisk up a month's supply of this shelf-stable, anti-aging moisturizer considered the equivalent of a world-famous beauty fluid.

3 tablespoons *each* honey and wheat germ oil

2 tablespoons *each* glycerin and witch hazel

1 tablespoon rose water

Place all ingredients in a glass bowl, whisk to combine, then store in a tightly capped bottle.

5

At-Home Facials with Salon-like Results

Prestigious salons, now catering to men as well as women, feature herbal steam treatments and natural masques based on formulas that have endured for centuries. At-home salon-type facials can be as sophisticated or as simple as is expedient. You can treat your face to a simple pack without any steamy preliminaries, have a two-minute hot-towel wrap, or indulge in a 10-minute steaming and a two-layer 30-minute masque.

Before You Begin: The "Bare" Essentials

Assembling the components is the first step. Charging out into the world in search of a fresh peach or a container of yogurt can be disconcerting when your pore-cleaned face is enhanced only with a towel turban. The next two steps are every-facial essentials:

1. Pull the hair back off your face with a ribbon or headband, or protect it with a wrapped-around towel.

2. Remove any makeup and cleanse your face as you would normally. Apply a moisturizer around your eyes and over your cheeks if your skin is exceedingly dry.

Facial Saunas: A Complete Guide to Cleansing, Purifying, and Softening Your Skin

Facial steaming improves circulation, softens roughness, clears out pores, and imparts a healthy glow to your plumped-up skin. The steaming can be a complete-unto-itself-facial if you follow it with a dousing of cool water or toner, then pat almost dry with a soft towel and smooth on moisturizer. For the ultimate in pore-flushing: the moment you finish steaming, close your eyes and spray your face with mineral water or toner. To incorporate a treatment with your spray:

- *For normal skin*: Mix camomile tea and cold skim milk half-and-half.

- *For dry skin*: Mix cold whole milk and rose water in equal proportions.

- *For oily skin*: Mix 1/3 cup triple-strength camomile tea with 2 teaspoons *each* lemon juice, skim milk, and witch hazel. Refrigerate the remainder to use as a toning refresher between steamings.

How to steam clean your skin

Steaming prior to applying a masque is optional; "opening your pores" is a matter of semantics. The American Medical Association states that pores are not controlled by muscles, therefore they cannot either open or close.[149] However, heat does affect the skin to allow free access to the pores and soften their contents. Barbershop hot-moist towels are a case in point. You can follow suit by wringing a lightweight towel out of hot water (with or without herbal enhancements), folding the towel lengthwise, and covering your face (except for nose and mouth) for two minutes. Electrical devices for releasing steam vapor have been used in Europe for over 50 years and are becoming increasingly popular in the United States, despite the fact that they have been charged with several cases of "jungle acne" resulting from overmoisturization.[32] If you have a facial sauna appliance, abide by its instructions. If you don't, there are no-cost methods of achieving similar results without the hazards. Be sure to keep your eyes closed, your face far enough away from the heat to avoid irritating your skin, and never steam for longer than 10 minutes.

To tent or not to tent (by draping a towel over your head to hold in the steam) is a question most experts answer in the affirmative. If you choose to tent, protecting your hair with a shower cap or towel turban before you cover up with the bath towel will prevent the aftermath of an overly curly or damply limp coiffure.

There are two options for do-it-yourself steaming: (1) Fill the bathroom basin with steamy-hot water and lean over it for 2 to 5 minutes. (2) If you wish to incorporate herbs to intensify the benefits, or if your tap water is not that hot, bring 1 or 2 quarts of water (plus herbs, if used) to a boil on the stove. Turn off the heat and either hover over the pot or move it to a table so you can sit comfortably for 5 to 10 minutes.

Herbal steaming supplements

Plain steam is good, particularly when you merely have blackheads to remove or wish to increase the effect of an exfoliant. Herbal steam is better and more penetrating for cleansing, purifying and softening. Use the same proportions as for making tea: one tea bag, or the equivalent in dry herbs or herbal oils, for each cup of water. For normal or combination skin, you can mix or match your favorite teas; for special effects, there are special suggestions.

- Acacia, clover, cowslip, elderflower, violet, and yarrow are recommended for dry skin.

- Camomile, eucalyptus, lavender, peppermint, and sage not only soothe and disinfect the skin (camomile is especially recommended for men and for everyone with blemished complexions), they contain aromatic oils beneficial to sinus passages.

- Elderflower, rosemary, and red dock root are suggested for steaming blackheads.

- Lemon, lemon grass, rose, and rosemary teas are especially helpful for oily complexions. To scent the house with lemon freshness while you purify your skin, simply add a few lemon slices to your simmering water and herbs.

- Vacation-simulating steam will rise nostalgically from a mixture of 1 tablespoon *each* camomile, eucalyptus leaves, juniper berries, and dry peppermint tea—or from pine needles or pine or bayberry oils. A tablespoon of kelp generates an oceanside tang.

Double-duty make-ahead herbal mixture for dry or normal skin:

1/4 cup *each* dried acacia flowers and elderflowers

1/4 cup *each* dried peach leaves and strawberry leaves

2 tablespoons *each* camomile, clover, lavender, and peppermint tea

2 tablespoons *each* crushed anise, caraway, and fennel seeds

2 tablespoons ground licorice root

Combine and store in an airtight container. When you are ready for a facial, place 2 tablespoons of the mixture in each quart of steaming water. For a masque to follow your steam cleaning: strain out the herbs, spread them on a washcloth moistened with the herbal water, then cover your face with the moistened cloth (herb-side-down) for 5 minutes.

Double-duty make-ahead herbal mixture for oily skin:

1/4 cup *each* camomile, lavender, lemon grass, and lemon peel

1/4 cup *each* dried peach leaves and strawberry leaves

2 tablespoons *each* crushed anise, caraway, and fennel seeds

2 tablespoons peppermint

Combine and store in an airtight container. For facial steaming: add 2 tablespoons of the mixture to each quart of boiling water. For a masque-after-steaming: strain out the herbs, spread them on a washcloth moistened with the hot liquid, then place the cloth (with the herbs next to your skin) over your face and let it remain until cool.

Stimulating steaming: How to give yourself the "hot and cold" treatment

To bring a glorious glow to a weary complexion, intersperse a cold-towel pack with your hot towels or hot-water-steaming. Place a few ice cubes in a bowl of cold water next to your steam source, saturate a towel in the ice water, then interrupt your steaming once each minute with a 20-second application of the cold towel.

Rosemary, sage, camomile and lavender (1 teaspoon of each) make a stimulating steam to help counteract a muddy or sallow complexion.

Natural Masques: How They Work, When to Use Them

Whether termed masques, masks, or packs, they dislodge cellular debris that can give skin a drab, gray cast, firm and clear skin, plump up wrinkles, and are the "fun" part of a facial. Mother Nature's line is more extensive and exciting than cosmetic-counter offerings, and far less costly. One budding-but-budgeting actress splurged on a "miracle masque," read the fine print on the gilt wrappings as the goo dried on her face, and was more than somewhat disappointed to discover that the product contained nothing more than egg white embalmed with preservatives, perfume, and artificial color. She could have filled her refrigerator with real eggs for the same price.

Intrepid experimenters report that masquing several times each day for months improves rather than harms their skin, and although few of us have time for such frequent indulgence, a brief facial pack before a breakfast meeting, or a 5-minute skin-tightening masque before a dinner engagement can be well worth the effort. Some dermatologists advise a twice-weekly steam treatment for women with average or oily skin, and for men who wear stage makeup or use bronzing gel. Most skin-care experts, however, suggest once a week for all men and women with normal skin, once a month for dry skin, and seldom if ever for those troubled by acne or spider veins because heat may aggravate either of these conditions.

Paying heed to the reaction of your own skin is the best guide to what is right for you. If your face is dry in some areas and oily in others, you may want to apply a different mask on each section (i.e., gelatin or avocado mixture for your cheeks, egg white for your T-zone). Although complexity and time requirements vary, the basic application and removal is similar for all:

1. With hair pushed back off your forehead, smooth or pat the masque over your entire throat and face except for the fragile skin around your eyes.

2. Allow the masque to dry thoroughly (5 to 30 minutes, 20 minutes is the accepted average). Reclining on a slantboard or lolling in bed with your feet propped on pillows and refreshing pads on your eyes while you listen to soft music is sensuously luxurious, and increases the benefits from a masque. Soaking in a scented tub prolongs drying time and enhances the masque's effect.

3. Remove the masque with warm or cool water, rinse well, then tone and moisturize.

Masquing Marvels That Rejuvenate and Nourish Your Skin

Prior steaming, or even a hot shower, will make your skin more receptive to a masque's nourishing treatment, but any of these masques may be applied to a freshly cleansed face.

Almond meal. Two tablespoons *each* almond meal, honey, and whole milk; blended and patted on, makes a masque for all skin types.

Cornmeal, mixed to a paste with egg white, smoothes rough, bumpy skin.

Eggs have been acknowledged skin beautifiers for centuries, probably since the first cavelady improved her appearance with a bit of pterodactyl egg. For all types of skin: Beat an egg until frothy; apply to the face, neck, and shoulders.

Eggnog masques. Each variation is ample for two (menfolk favor the alcoholic version) or for coating your shoulders, bosom, and face.

Cognac eggnog for normal or oily skin: Whisk (or whir in an electric blender) 1 raw egg with 2 tablespoons *each* cognac, lemon juice, and fluid milk. Let stand until room temperature before applying.

Alcohol-free eggnog for normal or dry complexions: Beat 1 tablespoon dry milk into a stiffly beaten egg white, then fold in an egg yolk stirred with 1 teaspoon honey.

Egg white, plain or beaten, smoothed on with the fingertips or applied with a blusher brush, pastry brush, or shaving brush, draws out impurities and refines the pores as it dries.

Egg white, beaten and mixed with 1 teaspoon honey, is a twice-a-day texturizer used by photographers' models. Let it dry on your skin for 10 minutes before rinsing off. Store the remainder in the refrigerator. For additional benefits, add 1 tablespoon of mashed papaya and the contents of a snipped vitamin-E capsule.

Egg-white and alum plus honey pack is an old-fashioned skin rejuvenator. Beat an egg white with 1/8 teaspoon alum, smooth on and let dry until your face feels very taut. Rinse thoroughly, blot dry, then pat on a coating of honey and let that remain for 5 minutes. Rinse off the honey and tone your face with rose water.

Egg white, milk, and honey skin tightener. Beat together 1 egg white, 1 tablespoon instant nonfat dry milk, and 1/2 teaspoon honey. Mint or sage tea is suggested as a toner after this masque has dried and been removed.

Egg yolk, lightly beaten with a fork, then smoothed on and allowed to dry, is a comfortably gentle skin firmer for dry or normal skin.

Egg-yolk honey is a masque for dry, wrinkle prone skin: Blend 1 egg yolk and 1 tablespoon honey with 1/4 teaspoon almond oil. Adding a tablespoon of yogurt makes it even more effective.

Egg yolk and olive oil, 1 teaspoon of the oil beaten with 1 egg yolk, is an Italian dry-skin treatment. For a variation with zing, blend the egg yolk with 2 teaspoons safflower oil and 1/2 teaspoon mint extract.

Fruit masques are easily prepared skin treats. (To rehydrate naturally dried, unsweetened fruit: soften in hot water or cook until tender.) Puree or mash enough fruit to cover your face and throat. Blend in 1 teaspoon oil, cream, or milk if your skin is dry or normal; 1 teaspoon lemon juice if your skin is oily or normal. For variety, try the following.

Apple. Originally developed as a masculine masque, this combination is equally effective for feminine faces. Core and quarter a small, unpeeled apple. Puree it in a food processor or electric blender with 1 tablespoon honey and 1/2 teaspoon dried sage (or 1 tablespoon snipped fresh leaves) for normal or combination skin; add 1 tablespoon lemon juice for oily complexions.

Apricots or peaches are valuable skin nourishers you can use as often as needed to refresh tired skin or enliven a wan complexion and make it less wrinkle prone. Blend in 1/2 teaspoon lemon juice with the pureed fruit before applying to oily skin; 1 teaspoon of cream, honey, or vegetable oil for dry skin. For a superlative skin-tightening masque, blender whir 1 egg white with the fruit.

Avocado, mashed or whirred in a blender with a few drops of lemon juice makes a nourishing, gently astringent masque for men or women. If your skin is very dry, add 1 egg yolk, or 1 tablespoon honey, or 1 teaspoon vegetable oil.

Banana, peeled and sliced or mashed, is a Guatemalan favorite for relieving dry skin. When you have time to lie perfectly still for 20 minutes, you can arrange thin slices of banana all over your face and let the banana's oils and vitamins permeate your epidermis. If you anticipate squirming or sneezing, mash the banana to a smooth paste before applying. For very dry skin, add 1 teaspoon olive oil while mashing the banana. For added benefits, incorporate the peel by blender-pureeing half a banana with half its peel (cut up) and 1 teaspoon honey.

Grapes cleanse and moisturize all types of skin. Whir a handful of seedless green grapes in an electric blender, smooth the puree over your face and throat, and wait 10 minutes before rinsing off. For a South American skin-rejuvenating treatment, blend a tablespoon of flour with the grape puree.

Melons—cantaloupe, honeydew, or watermelon, mashed or pureed—make a refreshing masque to cleanse and tighten pores and to help obliterate fine-line wrinkles.

Oranges are said to slow skin aging and erase signs of fatigue. Apply only the pulp, let dry for 15 minutes, remove with a damp washcloth and rinse thoroughly.

Papaya contains an enzyme, papain, which helps clear impurities and heal blemished skin. The peeled, mashed, or pureed fruit can be smoothed on, allowed to dry for 15 minutes, then rinsed off. For more exfoliating action: wait only 5 minutes after applying the papaya puree, gently massage your face with a fresh papaya slice, remove the melange with a washcloth, then rinse.

Pears, mashed or pureed with a bit of lemon juice, have astringent properties beneficial for oily skins.

Pineapple with honey is a tropical skin-texturizer. Smooth on a thin coating of honey and let dry for about 10 minutes, or until it feels tacky. Remove with cotton pads soaked in fresh pineapple juice, then apply a second coating of pineapple juice or rub a slice of fresh pineapple over your face. Wait a few minutes before rinsing.

Plums, cooked and mashed with a teaspoon of almond oil, make a rich 10-minute masque for oily skin.

Prunes do more than relieve costiveness, they can regenerate tired, dry skin. Blender-puree 4 cooked, pitted prunes with 1 teaspoon sesame oil.

Strawberries are time-tested skin improvers that clean pores, tighten skin, help clear up blemishes and postpone wrinkling. Mash fresh or frozen unsweetened strawberries, smooth the puree over your face, and let it dry for 10 minutes before rinsing off with cool water. For more pronounced cleansing and softening: Mix 1/4 cup mashed strawberries with 2 tablespoons cornstarch or yogurt; or blend the mashed strawberries with cream and/or oatmeal to make a pretty pink paste. This 10-minute after-shave masque is especially for men: 1 tablespoon mashed strawberries blended with 1 teaspoon sour cream.

Gelatin masques are ideal for dry or sensitive skin. Manufacture an easy one by softening a packet of unflavored gelatin in a little cold water, stirring the mixture over boiling water (or microwaving it) to dissolve, then letting it cool for a few minutes before smoothing over your face.

Yellow-Jell-O refresher. Dissolve 2 tablespoons lemon gelatin dessert in 1/4 cup boiling water, stir in 2 tablespoons strained fresh lemon juice, and let stand until room temperature.

Nourishing gelatin masque

1 teaspoon unflavored gelatin

1/4 cup water

1/4 cup soybean oil

1 tablespoon *each* liquid lecithin and sesame oil

1 teaspoon liquid multivitamins *or* 1 teaspoon *each* brewer's yeast and cod liver oil, the contents of a 100 IU vitamin-E capsule, and 1/4 teaspoon vitamin C crystals

Stir the gelatin into the water, heat to boiling, stir to dissolve, then pour into the container of an electric blender. Add all other ingredients and blend for 15 seconds. Apply and let penetrate for 10 minutes before rinsing off. Refrigerate the remainder for your next facial treatment.

Herbs. Any of the herbs or herbal combinations suggested for facial saunas may be steeped in boiling water, drained, and spread on a washcloth for use as a masque. For additional benefits, the herbs can be mixed to a paste with yogurt and/or lemon juice, then patted over the face.

Fresh bay or eucalyptus leaves, ground to a paste with regular-strength pekoe tea and allowed to stand for 24 hours, are a healing-toning masque recommended by plastic surgeons.[60]

Fresh mint refines pores when 1/4 cup of the leaves are blender-ground with 2 tablespoons almond meal and enough water to make a paste. Massage into your skin and let dry for 5 minutes. Rinse off; follow with a coating of honey; then let that dry for another 5 minutes before rinsing.

Pizza pack: Place 1 tablespoon dried Italian seasoning (from the spice shelf) in a cup with 1/4 cup tomato juice. Cover and let stand for 8 hours.

Honey, all by itself, is a stimulating, smoothing facial pack when patted on the face and allowed to remain for 5 minutes.

Honey and lemon juice is a French specific for lackluster skin. Mix 1 tablespoon honey with 1 teaspoon strained lemon juice. Apply to your freshly cleansed face and leave on for at least 30 minutes. Remove with rosemary tea or tepid water.

Honey and wheat germ, mixed to a paste, is another nourishing-masque option.

Mayonnaise, either store-bought or homemade (see Glossary for recipe), is a marvelous skin softener and revitalizer that can be used every day. Allow 5 to 20 minutes for it to permeate, then rinse off with warm water. For superbly smooth, rejuvenated skin: Mix 1 tablespoon mayonnaise with 2 teaspoons almond meal and 1/8 teaspoon alum.

Milk, like honey, not only contributes to other facials, but can masque alone. Skim milk aids oily skin; whole milk helps under-40 skin; half-and half or heavy cream discourages over-40 dryness; buttermilk cleanses and blanches; sour cream soothes dry skin; yogurt is good for every type of skin, has anti-bacterial properties, and helps thicken other masques.

Four-layer milk masque is a Hungarian treatment for delicate or dry skin. Mix a tablespoon of evaporated milk (or fluid whole milk) with 1/4

teaspoon of olive oil. Smooth a thin film over your skin with your fingers or a sponge, let it dry for a minute or two, then apply a second layer. Repeat until four layers have dried and your face feels like granite. Remove with lukewarm water and a washcloth.

Instant nonfat dry milk is a 5-minute skin-texturizer when mixed to a paste with water. If your skin is very dry, blend in a few drops of salad oil. If you want a pepper-upper, add 3 drops of peppermint extract. If you want to lighten as well as tighten your skin, use lemon juice to make the milk paste.

Sour cream is a soothing skin-tightener that first found favor with Russian czarinas.

Sweet cream or whipping cream soothes and texturizes dry skin.

Yogurt, plain or mixed with a few drops of lemon juice, makes a skin-toning pack. For a skin-lightening masque: Blender puree a slice of lemon and a quarter of an orange (both unpeeled) with 1/4 cup yogurt. Pat over your face and let dry for 20 minutes before rinsing off.

Milk of Magnesia, straight from the bottle, neutralizes the fatty acids that accumulate on oily skin. Simply smooth on, let dry for 15 to 20 minutes, then rinse.

Mud. If you don't have access to a natural spring surrounded by pure clay, you can pick up a package of fuller's earth at the corner drugstore. Mud or clay masques require 30 to 40 minutes drying time to clear off cellular debris, remove excess sebum from oily skin, and also lift out grime, blackheads, and whiteheads. If your skin type is dry or normal-combination, smooth on a protective film of salad oil before applying the masque. Mix the fuller's earth with mint tea, mint mouthwash, or witch hazel for extra zing.

Bret discovered a mud-masque bonus. Running late for a night meeting, he nicked his chin while shaving. With no time to spare, he covered the bleeding spot with a dab of the masque Jane had just prepared for her evening-alone beauty ritual. To their mutual surprise, the mud masque not only staunched the flow of blood; it also concealed all evidence of the mishap.

Alcoholic mud helps in treating super oily skin. Combine 2 tablespoons rubbing alcohol with 2 teaspoons fuller's earth. Add 1 teaspoon peppermint extract, if desired.

Almond mud is a cleansing-toning masque you can prepare by combining 1 tablespoon *each* almond meal and fuller's earth, a few drops of benzoin, and enough witch hazel to make a spreadable paste.

Carrot clay has blemish-healing as well as skin-texturizing qualities: Mix 1 tablespoon *each* carrot juice and fuller's earth with mineral water until you have a thick paste.

Egg-yolk mud sounds dreadful but does delightful things for dry or normal skin. Use a fork to beat 1 egg yolk with 1 tablespoon fuller's earth. Stir in 1 teaspoon honey and add mineral water to make a soft paste.

Herbal mud for oily skins can be prepared by steeping 1 teaspoon each rosemary and sage in 1/2 cup boiling water, straining, and mixing enough of the liquid with 2 tablespoons fuller's earth to make a smooth-on paste.

Muddy oatmeal is great for rejuvenating tired skin. Mix 1 tablespoon each leftover cooked oatmeal and fuller's earth with water to make a paste.

Yogurt mud refines pores and tightens normal or oily skin. Mix 1 egg white, 1 tablespoon yogurt, 1 teaspoon *each* fuller's earth and honey. Or, mix 2 tablespoons yogurt, 2 teaspoons fuller's earth, a few drops of mint extract, and enough water to make a creamy paste. Or, mix 1 tablespoon *each* yogurt and fuller's earth with 1/2 teaspoon honey and 1/8 teaspoon baking soda.

Oatmeal is given credit for many flawless complexions. Regular or quick-cooking dry oatmeal can be mixed with water or milk and allowed to dry on your face and throat for 10 to 15 minutes to smooth, soften, and remove dead cells. To multiply the benefits, blend 1 egg white, 1 tablespoon of instant nonfat dry milk, and 1/4 teaspoon almond oil with the oatmeal. For sensitive skin, pulverize the oatmeal in an electric blender or food processor; or stir 2 tablespoons oatmeal into 1/2 cup milk and cook it to soft mush.

For a spectacular dry-skin masque: Mix 2 tablespoons uncooked oatmeal with buttermilk or triple-strength camomile tea to make a thick paste. Or, mix 2 tablespoons *each* oatmeal and honey with 1 teaspoon white vegetable shortening. Or, mix 2 tablespoons oatmeal with 1 teaspoon *each* honey and cider vinegar, and 1/2 teaspoon almond meal.

Nutty Mexicali oatmeal improves circulation, conditions and feeds normal or oily complexions, but should not be used on dry or sensitive skin.

2 tablespoons *each* brewer's yeast, chopped cashew nuts, honey, and uncooked oatmeal

1 egg white

1/4 teaspoon chili powder

Place all the ingredients in the container of an electric blender. Whir until smooth, spread over your face and neck, and allow to dry for 30 to 45 minutes.

Oil packs are the original dry-skin remedy. Coat your face and throat with almond, olive, sesame, or wheat germ oil, or petroleum jelly; cover with a moist hot towel (leave your nostrils exposed); lie down until the towel cools. For even greater benefit, reheat and replace the towel several times. If you are ready for bed, just tissue off the excess oil; if not, remove it with warm water and a washcloth.

Sea spa masque. Mix sea salt with warm water until it is the consistency of moist sand. Pat over your face and let dry for 15 minutes, covered with a hot towel for the full effect. Aficionados claim this masque does more than rejuvenate the surface, it also shapes up droopy sags.

Vegetables are venerated beautifiers.

Beets make a magenta-hued masque that men and women will appreciate. In a blender or food processor, puree a raw beet with a teaspoon of heavy cream.

Carrots, grated, ground, or pureed in their raw state, help firm skin and clear blemishes. An exclusive strictly-for-males salon features a masque you can prepare in a blender from 1 tablespoon beer, 2 teaspoons *each* orange juice and grated carrot, 1 teaspoon yogurt, and 1/2 teaspoon lemon juice. If your skin is drier than the housemate with whom you are sharing, add a few drops of olive oil to your portion.

Cooking the carrots releases more of their vitamin A for added skin benefit. Mash them to a paste with a little of the unsalted water in which they were cooked; apply while still warm.

Corn, cut or grated from a fresh ear and mashed or pureed, is a soothing, toning masque for dry skin. Let the milky pulp dry on your face for 20 minutes.

Cucumber, blender-pureed with cream or yogurt, can work wonders for dry skin. For oily skin, blend a 2-inch chunk of peeled cucumber with an egg white or 2 teaspoons lemon juice plus 1/2 teaspoon mint extract. For normal-combination skin, add 2 teaspoons instant nonfat dry milk.

Peas, fresh or frozen, pureed in a blender and patted over face and throat, make a stimulating masque reported to help even out discolored patches of skin.

Penthouse Bunny Masque is concocted from "rabbit food" and may qualify your skin for a centerfold appearance: Blender-puree 1/4 cup *each* chopped cucumber, lettuce, and raw white potato with 1 lemon slice, 1/2 teaspoon dried peppermint, and 1/8 teaspoon vitamin C crystals. Scoop the mixture onto lettuce leaves, press over your face and throat, cover with hot-moist towels for 20 minutes, then remove with warm water.

Tomato is a mild astringent that refines pores and acts as an exfoliant. Cut a tomato in thin slices to place over your face for 10 minutes; or, drain the juice and seeds from the slices, mash them to a pulp and pat on. To add curative benefits for blemished skin: Mix in 1 teaspoon lemon juice plus a little brewer's yeast, oatmeal, and dry milk or yogurt. To increase penetration, cover the tomato masque with a hot, moist towel.

Wheat masques. For normal or oily complexions, mix raw wheat germ (or 1 tablespoon whole wheat flour) with 1/2 teaspoon vinegar plus water to make a paste. If your skin is dry, mix 1 tablespoon wheat germ with 1 tablespoon milk, yogurt or wheat germ oil. Let stand to soften before patting over your face, then extend the drying time by luxuriating in a beauty bath for 20 minutes.

Yeast. *Baker's yeast*, once sold in moist blocks or foil-wrapped cakes, is a perennial favorite for removing impurities and firming oily skin for males and females. Soften a packet of freeze-dried baking yeast in water to make a smooth paste, slather over your face, then let dry before rinsing off.

Brewer's yeast can be used for circulation-stimulating, texturizing masques. For normal or combination skin: Mix the yeast into a paste with water. For dry skin: Use milk as the liquid and add a teaspoon of honey; or incorporate 1 teaspoon *each* almond oil, honey, and lemon juice with 3 tablespoons brewer's yeast plus enough water to make a thick paste. For oily skin or normal-combination skin: Use rose water, witch hazel or yogurt to make a paste with the yeast. Add a few drops of peppermint extract for extra zing. For wrinkled skin: Use milk as the liquid and add the contents of a vitamin E capsule. If your skin is very dry, use wheat germ oil instead of milk to mix the paste. After the masque has dried and been rinsed off, rub a little of vitamin E oil (or wheat germ oil) into the wrinkled areas before retiring. For best results, apply twice weekly.

After the Facial Is Over:
How to Protect Your Salon-like Results

Scandinavians plunge into the snow after a sauna; you can give your facial a Finnish finish by splashing on cold water as the final rinse. To reestablish your skin's pH balance, apply your favorite toner or a mixture of one teaspoon cider vinegar or lemon juice and one-third cup water. Then, to seal in all the good things you have done for your now glowing and rejuvenated skin, apply a thin film of oil or your usual moisturizer.

❧ 6 ❧

Successful Strategies for Clearing Up Nagging Skin Problems

Skin is so closely related to emotional climate that it not only turns pale and clammy from anxiety, blushes in embarrassment, and glows with happiness; it also responds to malnutrition or stress, as well as external care. Complexion imperfections are equally distributed between the sexes and, for each problem, potential or existing, there are natural preventives and remedies.

Paraffin Heat Treatment:
Queen Nefertiti's Wax Secret Unmasked

Egypt's Queen Nefertiti is credited with originating this hot-wax facial which is now offered by twentieth-century salons as a multipurpose unisex skin clarifier and rejuvenator, and has been adapted for at-home use. If your skin is very dry, smooth a film of vegetable oil over your freshly cleansed face before beginning the treatment.

Melt half of a four-ounce cake of paraffin in a cup set in a pan of water over low heat. Test to be sure the wax is not hot enough to burn your skin, then paint your face—except for the tender area around your eyes—with a half-inch paintbrush. Apply generously so the wax forms an airtight seal.

55

Heat the back of a metal serving spoon by holding it close to water in your wax-melting pan; then "iron" your face with the spoon, paying particular attention to any blemishes, lines, or wrinkles the wax coating will have exaggerated. Continue the ironing for 5 minutes, reheating the spoon each time it cools.

Peel off the paraffin as soon as it solidifies after the ironing. Dry-skin lines or wrinkles will have softened and, if your face has been harboring impurities, they will have been drawn to the surface and embedded in the wax. Rinse with cool water, then apply your toner and moisturizer.

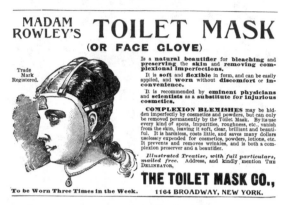

Madam Rowley's Face Glove must not have been as effective as promised; it vanished from the marketplace soon after this advertisement appeared in 1893.

How to Eliminate Blackheads and Whiteheads Safely and Naturally

Approximately 20 percent of the body's toxic waste is eliminated through the skin,[19] so scrupulous cleansing plus a diet containing a minimum of saturated fat is important for controlling and removing exterior accumulations of waxy oil. When a minuscule globule of sebum collects at the top of a pore, a whitehead develops; when the waxy oil hardens, plugs the pore and is exposed to air, it turns black through oxidation and becomes a blackhead. Called *comedones* by dermatologists, these facial pests can be exterminated by natural means.

Five home remedies for washing away blemishes

1. **Baking soda,** slightly moistened and gently massaged over whiteheads, is sufficiently abrasive to remove the thin covering so the sebum can escape.

2. **Almond meal.** Mix to a paste with water, work into the skin with a complexion brush, and rinse off with cool water.

3. **Cornmeal.** Blend half-and-half with white vegetable shortening, massage in, then tissue off before completely removing with soap and water.

4. **Soapy meal.** Combine 1/4 cup finely grated castile soap with 1/4 cup *each* almond meal and cornmeal; store in an airtight container. To use: scoop a spoonful of the mixture into the palm of your hand, moisten with water, and massage into your face with a complexion brush or sponge. Rinse thoroughly, then splash on a toner made from 1 teaspoon cider vinegar and 1/3 cup water.

5. **Tomato.** Even before "love apples" were deemed fit for human consumption, beauty-conscious damsels were instructed to cut a slice from one of the red orbs and rub it into areas plagued by "skin worms." (Tomato contains vitamin C plus an acid that removes dead epidermal cells, thus helping to clear whiteheads and prevent blackheads from turning into pimples.)

Removing blackheads—what the experts recommend

Squeezing is frowned upon by some dermatologists; others admit that physical force is the only way to dislodge deeply embedded blackheads and recommend using a "blackhead extractor" (a metal tool with a tiny hole in the end) or pressing out the offenders with tissue-wrapped fingertips. Before attempting either type of removal, soften the blackheads by steaming or with this "loosening solution" preferred by prestigious salons.

EPSOM SALT AND IODINE: Bring 1/2 cup water to a boil, stir in 1 teaspoon epsom salt and 3 drops of iodine. Dip strips of absorbent cotton in the slightly cooled solution, place them over infested areas and cover with a dry washcloth to retain the heat. Repeat two or three times, reheating the liquid if necessary. After popping out the blackheads, go over your face with peroxide or an alcohol-containing astringent.

How to Reduce Enlarged Pores

Usually resulting from the overactive sebaceous glands responsible for comedones, enlarged pores most often appear where the glands are most concentrated, such as on the nose, inner aspects of the cheeks, and the chin. Men are especially vulnerable to this problem, but, as all of us age, our skin loses elasticity and pore openings expand. Improving your diet by including more vitamin-A-containing foods (see the Vitamin and Mineral Chart), or augmenting with a supplement, may be helpful. (A deficiency of vitamin A can cause dead cells below the skin surface to clog oil glands and distend the delicate openings.) While nothing short of plastic surgery will permanently alter existing pore size, much can be done to make large pores less obvious.

- **Benzoin.** In the 1890s, men as well as women were advised to sponge their enlarged pores with a half-and-half blend of tincture of benzoin and water.

   Benzoin-cucumber lotion is an even more effective modern adaptation. Grate and mash (or whir in an electric blender) 1 cucumber. Strain into 1 cup of rose water and stir in 1 tablespoon tincture of benzoin. Refrigerate and apply with a cotton ball after each daily cleansing.

- **Buttermilk oatmeal.** Stir 2 tablespoons dry oatmeal into 1/4 cup buttermilk. Cover and let stand overnight. Strain off the liquid and smooth it over your face. Allow 20 minutes drying time, rinse off with cool water, rub with an ice cube, then blot dry.

   Buttermilk salt is easier to prepare. Make a gritty paste from buttermilk and table salt. Work into enlarged-pore areas, then rinse with warm water. Repeat several times a week.

- **Egg skin** is a poor-folks' pore-shrinker that also helps bring skin eruptions to a head. Break an egg, reserve its contents for other use, then carefully remove the membrane from the inside of the shell. Smooth this egg skin over the enlarged pores; let dry before peeling off.

- **Make-ahead pore reducer.** Pulverize half of a one-pound package of steel-cut oatmeal in an electric blender or food processor. Mix with 1/2 cup almond meal, 1/4 cup powdered orris root, and 1 ounce castile soap (grated from 4-ounce bar). Store in an airtight container. Whenever you cleanse your face, moisten 1 tablespoon of the mixture, apply gently with the fingertips, then rinse off.

How to Win the War Against Acne—And Protect Your Skin from Battle Scars

Papules and pustules sound, and are, ugly—but their eruption doesn't necessarily indicate acne. Facial blemishes can occur as a result of illness, emotional stress (witness pimples popping up before prom night or a promotional presentation), dietary indiscretions, or sketchy cleansing.

When sebum and dead skin cells seal up a pore-opening, the continuing flow of waxy oils may force the plug (a whitehead) to protrude as a blackhead, invade and inflame surrounding tissue, harbor bacteria, and erupt as an angry red bump. Pinching at a blackhead without removing it may also aggravate the skin into producing a blemish. The old rule, "never pick at a pimple," is still good advice; the infection may spread and scarring may result. The following treatments, old and new, for acne papules or pustules are equally viable for all pimples—masculine or feminine.

In true acne (*acne vulgaris*), cells in and around follicle openings reproduce at a greater rate than they die and are shed. Combined with excess sebum production triggered by hormones, the pore-clogged results are the scourge of more teenage boys than girls, and the bane of more women than men because of fluctuating hormonal levels due to menstrual cycles. "Allergy" acne, which can result from reaction to anything from facial cosmetics to the feathers in bed pillows, is no respecter of gender, and may appear on masculine chests and backs as well as faces.

Many men have found that giving their skin a mini-vacation by not shaving on weekends lessens acne-aggravating facial irritation; occasionally, however, more frequent shaving is the answer. Alan's acne, which he thought he'd outgrown, reappeared shortly after he began shaving. A dermatologist's examination revealed that each pustule contained, and was instigated by, an ingrown hair. Shaving more often, *with* instead of *against* the grain, resolved Alan's problem. Stubbornly resistant acne may require medical attention, but natural, at-home care usually is all that is needed.

How your diet can help reduce acne flareups

A balanced diet with adequate protein, ample fluids, sufficient vitamins and minerals, and enough fiber to avoid constipation is essential for basic skin health. Eating habits are no longer believed responsible for creating acne (theories regarding sexual activity, or its lack, as a cause have also been debunked), but nutrition, especially during breakout periods, plays as important role in its control. In their book, *Complete Handbook of Nutrition*,[118] Gary and Steve Null suggest two daily glasses of any combination of fresh carrot, cucumber, lettuce and/or spinach juice. Dr. Blaurock-Busch, co-author of *The No-Drugs Guide to Better Health*,[19] advises drinking one-half cup of beet juice (or eating steamed beets) twice each week. Dr. J. Daniel Palm[120] recommends that women substitute fructose for sugar a few days prior to the menses. Avoiding chocolate, nuts and other fatty foods, strong seasonings, and anything containing iodides (saltwater fish, shellfish, iodized salt, bromides) has benefitted some acne endurers. Personal experimentation is the best policy: eliminating all possible offenders for two weeks, then reintroducing them one at a time will let you know which foods trigger flareups.

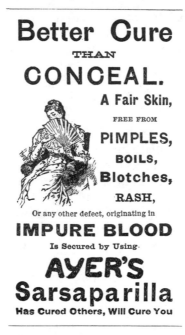
Herbalists advise drinking one or two cups a day of any one of these herb teas to "purify" the blood and clear skin disturbances: burdock, chaparral, chickweed, comfrey root, dandelion, red clover, strawberry leaf, valerian, white oak bark, or yellow dock.

Holistic doctors have found daily doses of up to 100,000 IU water-soluble vitamin A (for brief periods) and 5 grams vitamin C of benefit in some case of acne.[132] More impressive results have been obtained with the inclusion of a high-potency B-complex tablet, 400 IU vitamin D, 100 to 400 IU "dry" vitamin E, 1,000 milligrams calcium, and 50 milligrams zinc.[18,127] Acidophilus (in supplements or as a serving of yogurt with each meal) is often helpful and is considered essential whenever antibiotics are prescribed. Brewer's yeast or desiccated liver (one to two tablespoons, or the equivalent in tablets, daily) has proven effective for some individuals; and charcoal tablets (two after each meal for two weeks, then two per day) are credited with astounding results.[72]

Natural soapless cleansers

Gentle cleaning, performed several times daily to remove excess oil and surface contaminants, has been shown to successfully manage 25 percent of acne conditions.[132] Harsh scrubbing or the folk remedy of plastering pimply areas with soap and allowing it to remain overnight so irritates the skin that the sebaceous glands secrete even more sebum than they would normally. There are natural, soapless cleansers, but if you prefer soap and live in a hard-water area you can avoid the deposits of greasy sludge (created by soap mingling with water and minerals) by softening each quart of washing-rinsing water with one teaspoon of either baking soda or borax. Follow every cleansing with an astringent toner, then allow the pores to breathe by skipping the troubled areas when applying moisturizer.

- **Buttermilk or skim milk.** Wash your face with the milk, rinse with water, then reapply the milk and allow it to dry on your skin.
- **Lemon juice.** Dilute generously with water and rinse thoroughly.
- **Oatmeal, honey, and egg white.** Mixed to a paste and massaged into the face, this mixture cleanses the skin and loosens blackheads.
- **Rubbing alcohol.** Combine 1 part alcohol with 10 parts water.

Steam cleaning is seldom advised during acne outbreaks but brief steaming or hot-towel packs applied for a few minutes once or twice each day may coax the papules into vanishing, or may bring them to a head so they will open and drain.

Compresses, masques, poultices, and lotions

Unless otherwise directed, follow each of these natural treatments with a tepid-water rinse and an application of 3-percent hydrogen peroxide, a solution of one tablespoon vinegar and half a cup of water, or an astringent.

- **Aloe vera gel and lecithin.** Whir 1/4 cup aloe vera gel with 1 tablespoon water-soluble lecithin powder in an electric blender. Apply once each day and let remain for at least 15 minutes, preferably several hours or overnight, before rinsing off. Use plain aloe vera gel as a moisturizer for your entire face.

- **Bran and baking soda.** Mix 1 tablespoon miller's bran and 1 teaspoon baking soda to a paste with water. Pat over your skin and rinse off after 15 minutes.

- **Cabbage.** You can prepare a lotion by liquefying enough raw cabbage to make 1 teaspoon of "juice" and mixing it with an equal amount of tincture of benzoin. It smells terrible but helps clear blemishes.

- **Cabbage pack.** Soften cabbage leaves in hot water with a pinch of boric acid. Spread the leaves over your face and let them remain for 20 minutes.

  White cabbage pack, consisting of nothing more exotic than the ground or mashed inner leaves of raw cabbage, is a German treatment for skin blemishes.

- **Carrot pulp,** blender-pureed from raw carrots or mashed from cooked ones, improves broken-out skin when thickened with instant nonfat dry milk, patted on and allowed to dry.

- **Cornstarch and alcohol.** Mix rubbing alcohol with a teaspoon of cornstarch to make a paste. Dab a bit on each pimple with a cotton-tipped swab, leave in place for 30 minutes to 8 hours before rinsing off.

Gerald had wonderful success with this drying-out remedy suggested by his barber; his occasional pimples disappeared after a few overnight treatments. Suddenly, however, the pustules began multiplying so noticeably that the barber asked if he had been trying a new treatment. "No, I'm still daubing on the cornstarch and alcohol every night," Gerald said. "The only thing 'new' is the shaving brush I bought last month. First time I've ever used one, and, if it wasn't for these pimples, I'd really enjoy shaving every morning." After the barber explained that shaving brushes can become contaminated with bacteria from existing pustules and spread the infection, Gerald went back to lathering up with his hands. By the time he went in for his next haircut, the acne was once again under control.

- **Cucumber and rum.** Blend 2 tablespoons grated raw cucumber with 2 teaspoons rum. Pat on and let dry before rinsing. Refrigerate the remainder to apply as the next treatment.

- **Dock root,** also called yellow dock, is a centuries'-old cure for skin eruptions. You can mash the hot, cooked, roots, spread them on gauze squares and apply them to your face for 30 minutes (replacing the compresses when they cool); or blender-puree the dock with the water in which it was cooked, strain, and use the liquid as a clearing-toning lotion each time you wash your face.

- **Eggs.** Smooth on a film of vitamin E (from a pierced capsule), wait 30 minutes, then apply a coating of whisked egg white.

  Egg yolk, despite its fat content, often brings improvement when lightly beaten, patted over the skin, and allowed to dry.

- **Garlic.** Rub a slice of fresh garlic over the pimples several times each day.

- **Honey.** Use plain or mix with raw wheat germ to kill germs and draw out blemishes. Apply with tapping motions, wait 5 minutes before rinsing off.

- **Milk of magnesia** is not only a "drawing" masque, it is, according to makeup expert Paula Begoun,[12] a more effective acne medication than those prescribed by doctors. Smooth over your clean skin, let dry, then rinse off. Repeat several times daily but never leave on your face overnight.

- **Oatmeal.** Cook in milk and apply daily as a 10-minute masque.

- **Papaya mint tea**, brewed double strength and applied as a hot compress for 15 minutes twice daily, often brings immediate improvement and clears skin within two or three days.[32]

- **Pears** have a disinfectant, drawing action when peeled, cored, mashed, and used as a 10-minute facial pack.

- **Potato lotion.** Grate a raw potato into a sieve over a bowl and let stand until the "juice" drips out. Apply this liquid with a cotton ball, let dry before rinsing.

- **Tomato pulp** helps heal blemishes. Mash or puree tomato slices and blend with nonfat dry milk to make a paste. Smooth on and let dry for 10 minutes.

- **Valerian tea.** Prepare double strength and apply as a hot compress several times a day.

- **Witch hazel.** Saturate gauze or cotton pads with witch hazel straight from the bottle, and cover the affected areas for 5 minutes at a time at least once a day.

Sunlight

Exposure to the sun helps kill pimple-causing germs on the skin, instigates the body's production of vitamin D to assist with the assimilation of skin-improving vitamin A, and encourages the upper epidermal layer to peel off and unplug the oil-gland ducts. Moderation is essential, however, to prevent provoking a pimply condition with a sunburn or with the mineral salts from perspiration. If you're using an acne medication containing retinoid acid, be forewarned that when exposed to ultraviolet light it can increase the danger of burning and the risk of skin cancer. A 60-watt light bulb in an unshielded base offers an alternative to sunlight. It won't do anything for your vitamin-D supply, but, when positioned a foot away from the pustules for 15-minute periods, may help dry them up.

All-Natural Treatments for Dealing with Skin Discolorations

Acne rosacea: The red-faced flush

No respector of skin type or sex, acne rosacea's red-faced flush is aggravated by extreme temperatures, emotional stress, eating highly spiced foods, or imbibing alcoholic beverages. In severe cases, more common among men than women, small acne-like pimples appear and the skin may thicken, become purplish-red over the cheeks and chin, and create the bulbous-looking nose associated with chronic alcoholism. Usually, however, the dilated blood vessels responsible for the unattractive rosiness will shrink back to normalcy with proper care.

Here are some preventive measures you can take:

- Protect your face from inclement weather, wind, and fireplace or open-oven-door heat.

- Cleanse gently with mild cleansers and tepid water. Use non-tingly toners or after-shave lotions; refrain from exfoliating scrubs, facial saunas, or icy chillers.

- Eat and drink wisely. Supplement your daily multivitamin with a B-complex tablet at each meal; up to 300 milligrams per day of each of the "major" Bs is considered safe for periods of a few weeks. [107] (Alcohol destroys vitamin B, which may account for acne rosacea being dubbed "grog blossoms" in colonial times.)

Blotchiness

In addition to the treatments described for dealing with a fading tan in chapter 9, ingesting two tablespoons of brewer's yeast daily, including fresh peas and fish in your diet, and frequently splashing your face with a solution of one tablespoon vinegar plus one-half cup water, may help obliterate the blotchiness. Masques of mashed fresh peas or raw wheat germ blended with honey have also proven beneficial.

Spider veins

Fair skins are most susceptible to these little red lines (technically termed *telangiectases*) that wander over cheeks and noses, but anyone can acquire them from a variety of causes. Overzealous scrubbing or black-head squeezing, dilation from overexposure to sunlight, or the sudden contraction and expansion necessitated by wintery cold and indoor heat may rupture close-to-the-surface capillaries. Vitamin deficiencies can so weaken them that blood seeps out into surrounding areas and/or they lose their elasticity. With tender care, the tiny veins become less obvious and may shrink back into oblivion. The *don't*s are the same as those for acne rosacea: avoid irritation from extreme temperature changes, harsh physical treatment, or overindulgence in spicy foods or alcohol. The *dos* are also similar, with a few additions.

FOODS AND SUPPLEMENTS: To augment your basic good-skin diet (sufficient protein, lots of fiber-rich fruits and vegetables, ample fluid), take a multivitamin-mineral and at least one B-complex tablet each day. To strengthen capillaries and connective tissues, eat foods high in vitamin C (see the Vitamin and Mineral Chart) and take supplements of C plus bioflavinoids.

HERBAL TREATMENTS:

- **Camomile and white oak bark:** Simmer 1/2 teaspoon white oak bark in 1 cup water for 10 minutes, add 1/2 teaspoon camomile, turn off the heat and let stand, covered, until comfortably warm. Strain. Saturate pieces of cotton cloth in the liquid and place them over the veins for 5 minutes at a time once each day.

- **Parsley:** Cook half a bunch of freshly washed parsley in water to cover, or whir the raw parsley and water in an electric blender. Strain. Stir a teaspoon of honey into the liquid and smooth it over the spidery veins several times a day.

- **Shave grass:** This is a folk remedy for alleviating splotchy veins and improving the elasticity of connective tissue. Place 2 teaspoons dried shave grass in 1 cup cold water. Bring to boiling, cover and let steep for 10 minutes before straining. Drink two-thirds of the tea, then saturate cotton cloth in the remainder and cover the affected area for 5 minutes. Repeat the treatment every other day.

How to Perk Up Pale Faces

Medieval beauties aspired to skin so pale that a swallow of red wine could be seen flowing down their throats. This about-to-faint look is no longer desirable. If your physician has verified that your wan appearance is not due to internal dysfunction, you can restore a healthy glow by:

- Exfoliating your face every few days to dispense with dead-cell debris and revive natural color.

- Getting more fresh air and exercise to stimulate your circulation.

- Getting more rest and sleep to counteract the exhaustion that might be responsible for your weary appearance.

- Icing the skin surface to stimulate blood flow. If you are not troubled with broken veins, crush a few ice cubes, wrap them in a thin towel, spritz with witch hazel from a spray bottle, then rub the frosty bundle over your face and throat with uplifting motions. Repeat several times a week.

- Rubbing a cube of fresh watermelon over your face and letting the liquid dry before rinsing. (You can stash a cache of small chunks of watermelon in a plastic bag in the freezer for retrieval during out-of-season months.)

- Masking your face with soy powder and yogurt mixed to a paste, rubbed in and allowed to remain for 30 minutes before removing with a wet washcloth.

- Supplementing your diet with copper, folic acid, and iron (see the Vitamin and Mineral Chart for food sources).

- Trying the folk-healers' advice for "pallid women": Bathe your face in water to which a few drops of tincture of benzoin have been added. If this is not sufficient, follow with an application of 1/8 teaspoon benzoin mixed with 1 tablespoon rose water and allow it to dry on the skin. If all else fails, mix 1 tablespoon rose water with 1/2 teaspoon each ammonia and glycerin, rub into your face after the benzoin wash, let dry for 3 minutes, then blot with a soft towel.

How to Smooth Rough, Bumpy Skin

Sometimes appearing as "goose flesh" on the backs of upper arms as well as on male and female faces, small bumps at the base of invisible hair follicles are called *folliculosis*. They, and rough-textured skin, may indicate a deficiency of Vitamin A that can be corrected by daily supplements of 25,000 IUs of A plus 400 IUs of vitamin D. Here are some other suggestions:

- Facial scrubs and steams help to depose any accumulation of dead cells or pore-clogging soil which might be responsible for the roughness.
- Pat on some honey and allow a few minutes of skin-softening-time before rinsing off.
- Massage mayonnaise (store-bought or made from the recipe in the Glossary) into your face, let permeate for 5 minutes or leave on as a skin-smoothing night cream.
- Rose water and brandy, combined half-and-half and sponged over the face several times daily, is an 1890's suggestion for combating windburn or persistent roughness.
- Rosemary egg white is a skin smoother that should be stored in the refrigerator and applied every other day: Steep 1 teaspoon dried rosemary in 2 tablespoons boiling water for 15 minutes. Strain, then blend with 1 egg white and 1 teaspoon instant nonfat dry milk.
- Watercress water is a time-proven remedy for rough skin. Boil a cup of freshly rinsed, chopped watercress leaves and stems in a cup of distilled water. Let cool, strain, and apply several coats of the liquid. Allow each layer to dry before the next application, then rinse with cool water. Store in the refrigerator and use daily until improvement is noticeable. Prepare a fresh supply every seven days and continue biweekly treatments as preventive maintenance.

~ 7 ~

Managing Maturing Skin: How to Help Offset— & Prevent—Unsightly Lines, Sags, & Wrinkles

No one wants the expressionless face of an android or a store manikin; the goal is to maintain a youthful appearance by postponing or lessening the lingering lines from smiles and scowls that herald what we regard as "maturing skin." Our adversaries are the biological reduction of glandular activity which dries skin and deteriorates its connective tissues so lines and wrinkles form; and gravity, whose downward pull creates baggy eyes, saggy jowls, and double chins. Mother Nature is the ally who will assist our nurturing efforts, diminish the signs of time, and slow their advance.

Tips on Nourishing Maturing Skin

What you ingest affects facial muscles and supportive tissues as well as the epidermal surface. To compensate for the body's gradually slowing cell production and less efficient metabolism of foods, it is important to provide it with ample protein (meats, eggs, dairy products, legume-grain-milk combinations), and with a generous supply of vitamins.

Manufacturers offer higher-potency multiples for the "chronologically advantaged"; nutritionists often advise adding individual supplements:

- Taking a daily B-complex tablet (and/or a tablespoon or so of brewer's yeast) is good insurance. Laboratory tests have shown that a deficiency of any one of the Bs causes young animals to develop the wrinkled aspects of old age.[74]

- Vitamin C is good for collagen and elastin, the intertwining fibers supporting your face. Collagen cannot be absorbed from even the most convincingly advertised cosmetic, it is produced and maintained by the body from ingested protein and vitamin C with the assistance of the B complex.[149] Taking 1,000 to 5,000 milligrams of vitamin C in divided doses each day helps preserve and rejuvenate collagen's ability to prevent lines, sags, and wrinkles.[7]

How to Control Expression Lines

The 55 muscles in your face, each "wired" to nerves connected to your brain, react to everything you do, eat, or think. Except for those around your eyes and mouth, these muscles are not bound to the bones as they are on the rest of the body; they are attached to the skin by wisps of fibrous tissue that gradually lose their elasticity and allow your skin to become set in its ways. Facial tenseness, squinting, frowning in concentration or displeasure all pull at the skin, bunching it up to create little furrows which can become permanent expression lines. Although considered "character lines" on masculine faces, they are an aging-skin giveaway men as well as women are eager to postpone. These lines are so commonplace that remedies abound. Facial massage, gently performed on clean, lubricated skin is one solution. Isometric exercises are considered ideal for improving facial muscles (laboratory tests show that tensing muscles for six to ten seconds each day increases their resistance to our expression lining and gravity's efforts[132]). Smoothing out the lines with surface reminders is another option.

"Label" your lines

Trim stationery-store gummed or peel-and-press labels to fit your lines. Cleanse and dry your face, then gently rub the lines against the grain to flatten the skin before pressing the label in place. For normal training, leave in place for 30 minutes at a time, three times a week. For an accelerated course, sleep with your labels one or two nights a week. Peel off carefully (after moistening mucilage-backed labels), rinse with warm water, then use your toner and moisturizer.

Learn to watch yourself

Keeping a mirror by your telephone is a tricky way to catch yourself frowning or wrinkling your brow as you talk. Once you are aware of how these expressions "feel" on the inside, you can avoid them.

Smiling at yourself also pays handsome dividends. You have to experiment. You don't want to look like Mona Lisa or the Cheshire Cat—just a hint of a smile. After you practice for a while, it becomes automatic.

Psychocosmetics: Do-It-Yourself Physical and Mental Face Control with the Help of a Mirror

Based on the premise that radiant external beauty can be developed through physical and mental face-control in front of a mirror, Psychocosmetics is a European science you can practice without a license.

1. Slowly bend your head backward, then forward until your chin touches your chest. Relax your lower jaw and shake your head for a minute.
2. Raise your head, place your palms over your cheeks, and bend your head back as far as possible for a few seconds.
3. Lift your head, look yourself in the eye (in the mirror), and give your facial muscles some positive autogenic suggestions: "The corners of my mouth rise, my forehead is smooth" . . . whatever reinforcement your face may require. Conclude the treatment with a deep yawn.

Relaxing your face

1. Lean back, tense your face by squinching your eyes shut and clenching your teeth, then relax. Imagining warm water flowing over your face may assist relaxation efforts. Relaxing your hands by shaking them vigorously before dropping them limply in your lap also encourages facial relaxation.

2. Mentally visualize yourself in a calmly pleasant setting. Once you establish this feeling of untensed muscles, maintain it for five minutes by luxuriating in your imagination and rejecting any interfering, stressful thoughts; then yawn deeply.

Flattening forehead and frown lines

1. Banding your forehead increases circulation and helps break unconscious habits of brow wrinkling. Make your headband by sewing or pinning a 3-inch-wide elastic bandage so it fits snugly. Prepare a medicated lotion by dissolving 1/4 teaspoon epsom salt in 1 tablespoon hot water, then stirring in 2 teaspoons glycerin and 1 teaspoon 10-percent menthol solution. Use a cotton ball to smooth the liquid over your forehead, position the band, and leave it in place for an hour once each day.

2. Massaging, plumping or stroking minimizes both horizontal and vertical lines. Sit with your elbows resting on a tabletop, apply cream or oil to your forehead.

   Massage by pressing your left hand firmly on the hairline on the right side, then using the fingertips of your right hand to rub the area below your left hand with circular motions for 10 seconds. Move your left hand to the center of your hairline, then to your left side, repeating until your entire forehead has been massaged.

   Plump by creating suction between the heel of one hand and the lines, then vigorously "pumping" at least 10 times.

   Stroke your forehead gently, with upward-outward motions starting between your brows, until you feel a soothing sense of relaxation.

3. Exercising your forehead requires working the muscles against resistance because there is such a thin layer of tissue supporting the skin.

   a. Press the heels of your hands against each temple. Intermesh your fingers over your forehead, hold them stationary while attempting to first pull your forehead up toward your hairline, then down toward your eyes. Maintain each position for 10 seconds, repeat 5 times.

   b. Press the heel of one hand over your scowl lines to flatten them out. Try to move the skin by attempting to frown against the pressure, then try to stretch the frown muscles toward your temples. Repeat each movement 5 times.

Negating nose to mouth furrows

Exercise can help avoid or abolish the parenthesis-shaped lines between nose, mouth, and cheeks.

1. Puff out your cheeks as far as you can, then use your fists to press out the air. Repeat 10 times.

2. Simulate a kiss by puckering your lips. Move them in a circle from right to left, then left to right. Repeat 8 times for each side. Follow by opening your mouth wide, then puckering up again. Repeat 10 times.

3. Smile toothlessly by slowly opening your mouth and turning the corners up as you keep your teeth covered with your lips. Hold until you experience tension, then slowly form an "O" with your mouth. Relax and repeat.

4. Squeeze your eyes shut, wrinkle up your nose, hold for 10 seconds. Relax, then repeat 10 times.

- Masque the furrows. To decrease line depth, make a thick paste of brewer's yeast and water. Pat it over the lines and let dry. Rinse off with warm water, blot, then smooth on moisturizer. Repeat 3 times each week.

- Soften the lines by massaging them with a dab of moisturizer each time you cleanse your face.

How to Safely Minimize Wrinkles

Product-promises for producing more youthful skin probably predate Cleopatra, but none, so far, has proven reliable. *The Harvard Medical School Health Letter* of December 1987 states that estrogen-containing cosmetics have no long-lasting results; and the anti-wrinkle food supplement *SOD* (superoxide dismutase) can't even reach the skin because its enzymes are destroyed by digestive juices in the stomach.[21] The exciting news about wrinkle-removing *tretinoin* (a derivative of vitamin A marketed as Retin-A) has been tempered by the results of further study; the *University of California, Berkeley Wellness Letter* (April 1988) reports that four months of treatment were required before even subtle improvements were apparent, and that most of the subjects tested suffered skin inflammation lasting from two weeks to several months. *Alpha hydroxy acids* are another recently unveiled "fountain of facial youth." *Prevention* (March 1988) describes these acids as natural compounds which, when used under the guidance of a dermatologist, can change the structure of the skin to reduce existing wrinkles. While waiting for these miraculous cures to be perfected, there are many natural methods for regenerating our maturing faces.

Three ways to revitalize dry skin

Heredity is only one factor in the onset of after-30 dryness and lack of resiliency besetting most women and many fair-skinned men. Exposure to ultraviolet rays or smoking (which impairs circulation by constricting blood vessels) hastens the process. You can forestall drying, collagen collapse, and premature wrinkling by:

- Humidifying your rooms during the heating season to add moisture to your skin's environment.

- Including two tablespoons of unsaturated oil in a balanced diet containing adequate protein; counting your drinks to be sure you imbibe the equivalent of six to eight glasses of water each day; and taking a daily multivitamin-mineral supplement, a B-complex tablet, and at least 1,000 milligrams of vitamin C (more, if you smoke).

- Pampering your skin with gentle cleansers, toners, moisturizers, and masques, including this herbal-oil treatment: Empty the contents of 2 camomile tea bags into a jar. Add 1/4 cup sesame oil and 2 tablespoons wheat germ oil. Shake to combine, let stand for 24 hours. Shake again, strain the oil, and store it in the refrigerator. Smooth over dry-skin areas after your morning cleansing, let permeate for 5 minutes, then rinse off with luke-warm water. Repeat before bedtime, but instead of rinsing, blot the excess oil with a tissue and leave the remainder for an all-night treatment.

Eight wrinkle-prevention treatments

Cheeky is what wrinkles are, and where they usually make their first appearance. As reported in *University of California, Berkeley Wellness Letter* (February 1989) women are more prone to wrinkling than men because most males have a thicker dermis (the layer just under the skin's surface), which remains elastic longer than a woman's. Sleeping on your back to avoid skin-tugging-and-wrinkling by your pillow is one method of prevention and treatment, and there are others:

- Castor oil, cocoa butter, and coconut oil, the most revered wrinkle chasers, may be applied as frequently as desired.

- Eggwhite. Daily use of any of the eggwhite masques described in chapter 5, or merely covering your face with raw egg white (with or without a few drops of lemon juice) each morning before you brush your teeth and rinsing it off as you shower, can produce dramatic results.

- Egg yolk and mayonnaise. Use a "blush brush" to paint your face with raw egg yolk, applying it thickly over wrinkled or lined areas. While the egg is drying, mix 2 tablespoons mayonnaise with 1/2 teaspoon *each* fuller's earth and powdered kelp. Apply this paste over the egg yolk; rinse off after 10 minutes.

Mayonnaise, bottled or homemade (see Glossary for recipe), has transformed "prune faces" into "peaches and cream" when applied several times daily for several months.[40] For speedier results, blend an egg yolk with 1/4 cup of the mayonnaise.

- Ironing out the wrinkles is a before-the-party treatment. Cleanse your face, smooth on a generous coating of petroleum jelly or vegetable oil, then "iron" the lines and wrinkles with the bowl of a metal spoon heated in a cup of hot water. Go over your face several times, reheating the spoon when it cools. Tissue off the excess oil and sponge your face with a mild freshener.

- Lecithin granules, dissolved in warm water, mixed with cold-pressed vegetable oil and rubbed into the skin for all-day or all-night treatments reduce wrinkles when used religiously over a period of months.

- Oatmeal masques soften skin, making it less prone to wrinkle. For a no-bother, daily regimen: Reserve 1/4 cup leftover breakfast oatmeal in the refrigerator. Every evening, mix 1 tablespoon of the oatmeal with 1/2 teaspoon each cream and vegetable oil. Gently massage over your face and throat, and rinse away after 20 minutes.

- Olive oil, lemon juice, and salt improve skin as well as salad. Twice each day, rub olive oil into your clean face. Pat on lemon juice, drop by drop, until your skin feels "tacky," then briskly rub sea salt (or a half-and-half blend of epsom salt and table salt) over your face. Rinse off with warm water and blot dry.

- Yogurt and Vitamin E are aging-skin fighters. Blend 2 teaspoons yogurt and 1/2 teaspoon *each* honey and lemon juice with the contents of a 400 IU vitamin-E capsule. Smooth over your face, let penetrate for 15 minutes, then rinse.

Egg white: Nature's unique wrinkle-eraser

Egg white can make wrinkles disappear for a few hours. Stir a raw egg white with a fork, then use a fine camel's hair brush to carefully paint each visible wrinkle. For around-the-eyes lines, pat on a thin-as-possible coating of the egg white. Let dry, then apply a makeup foundation with equal care, using tapping rather than stroking motions.

Tom watched Martha painting our her wrinkles and was so astounded by the results he decided to try egg white on the fine lines around his eyes. Rather than resort to painstaking brush strokes, he simply rubbed his finger around the inside of an eggshell, then smoothed on the thin film of egg white. The effect was almost instantaneous. Now, each time Martha cracks an egg, Tom applies his wrinkle eraser.

Coping with Crow's Feet

- **Exercise** tones muscles to prevent or diminish crow's feet and eye crinkles.

  1. Open your eyes as wide as possible. Look up, down, to the left, and to the right, holding each position for 6 seconds.

  2. Close your eyes, scrunch up your face, and hold that position for 6 seconds. Then open your eyes and raise your eyebrows for 6 seconds.

  3. Place your palms on your cheeks, your fingers at the outer corners of each eye. With the fingers, draw the eye muscles toward your temples. Hold for 6 seconds, relax, then repeat.

- **Massage** stimulates circulation to strengthen muscles and revitalize skin. Without stretching the skin, run your fingers around the bony edge of your eye sockets. Begin at the bridge of the nose, move under the eyebrows, then across the top of the cheeks. Repeat until you have made 6 complete trips around your eyes. To stimulate the under-eye area, fingertip-tap the circular area from the top of your ears to the bridge of your nose.

- **Vitamin E.** Doctors Evan and Wilfred Shute[156, 157] who pioneered vitamin E research, discovered that alpha tocopherol molecules penetrate the epidermis to reach supporting skin tissues, and demonstrated that when applied regularly, vitamin E's firming and tightening action postpones and lessens wrinkles. Independent clinical studies verify that four weeks of under-eye treatment with vitamin E can make fine lines less noticeable.[45]

  Snip a capsule of d-alpha tocopherol (not a "dl" synthetic or "mixed" tocopherol). Pat the slightly sticky liquid under your eyes and let it dry. If your treat your face twice a day, use 200 IU capsules; if only once each day, use 400 IU capsules.

De-lining Your Mouth: How to Offset Surrounding Lines

A variety of remedies are offered for abolishing, or at least reducing, vertical or cross-hatched lines between the upper lip and nose, and the tiny crevices that cause lipstick to bleed into skin surrounding the mouth. Patience is a necessary virtue in these treatments; it took years for the "whistle marks" to develop, and it may take months to reduce or obliterate them.

- Vitamin E (from a snipped capsule), or wheat germ oil, sometimes dispenses with these sunburst lines when rubbed across-the-grain to flatten and fill in cracks and crevices.
- Do-it-yourself skin peels, performed twice weekly on the area between nose and upper lip, help smooth out these lines. Experiment with the exfolients in Chapter 2; or heat a tablespoon of bottled mineral water, stir in 1/2 teaspoon sea salt, rub it in and let it dry, then rinse off and follow with a moisturizer.
- Exercises are especially effective around the mouth because the muscles are directly attached.

  1. Form an "O" with your mouth. Tense the muscles for 6 seconds. Relax for 6 seconds. Repeat 5 times.

  2. Open your mouth as wide as possible by simulating a yawn, then pull your lips over your teeth and smile toothlessly. Hold for 6 seconds, relax, then repeat 5 times.

  3. Push your lips out as far as possible and suck in your cheeks. Hold for 6 seconds, then relax. Repeat 5 times.

Firming Up: How to Sabotage Gravity's Sags and Bags

Movie makeup artists pad young faces with wads of cotton to portray aging visages. In real life, gravity and flabby muscles produce the bulgy sags, while firming the muscles with massage and exercise preserves (or restores) youthful contours. In addition:

- Apply creams or oils with upward strokes on the face and with gentle taps around the eye area to avoid pulling or stretching the fragile skin.
- Munch chewy nibbles such as carrot and celery sticks to improve your jawline as well as your middle.
- Eat a well-balanced diet to provide Mother Nature with the ingredients for cell production, and don't succumb to yo-yo

dieting which can shrink and stretch skin tissues almost beyond repair.

- Recline on a slant board for a few minutes each day to reverse gravity's pull and increase blood circulation to the face.

How to massage your face and throat

Giving yourself a facial massage is fundamentally a matter of lubricating your skin and working your way up from throat to forehead with firm-but-gentle movements. Skin specialists advise a more precise method of manipulating your face after you have coated it with petroleum jelly, vegetable oil, or either of these two lotions to help your fingers glide over the skin.

Almond-castor oil lotion: In a wide-mouth jar, combine 1/4 cup *each* almond and castor oil with 2 tablespoons petroleum jelly and 1/2 teaspoon peppermint extract (optional). Refrigerate if it is not all used within 2 weeks. Warm in a pan of hot water if it becomes too thick to spread.

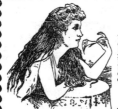
GINSENG-GELATIN LOTION

1/2 cup bottled mineral water (divided)

1 teaspoon unflavored gelatin

1-1/2 teaspoons ginseng powder or crushed ginseng tablets

1/2 teaspoon *each* glycerin and powdered kelp

1 capsule *each* natural vitamin A and vitamin E

Place 3 tablespoons of the mineral water in the container of an electric blender. Sprinkle with the gelatin and let it soften while bringing the remainder of the water to a boil. Pour in the hot water and whir to blend. Add remaining ingredients—squeezing in the contents of the capsules—and blend on medium speed. Decant into a wide-mouthed jar and refrigerate if not used within a week or so.

Here's how to massage your face and throat:

1. Pull your hair away from your face with a headband or towel turban. Sit comfortably at a table and rub a generous amount of your massage lotion between your palms.

2. Point your chin toward the ceiling. Using rapid strokes, smooth your palms upward and outward from collarbone to chin on each side of your neck. Repeat 5 times. Then apply lotion to the heel of one hand and use it to massage the tensed muscles under your chin.

3. Starting at the chin line on either side of the mouth, lift upward and outward from mouth to cheekbone, using your palms with firm, gliding motions. Repeat 10 times.

4. Apply lotion to the backs of your fingers. Make a fist with each hand and use your coated fingers to make firm, upward movements from your jawline to the tops of your ears. Repeat 10 times.

5. Dip your fingertips in the lotion. Place your fingers in the center of your forehead and sweep toward the temples. Repeat 10 times. Arch your fingers and press the entire forehead from brow to hairline, allowing 5 seconds for each pressure area. Follow by firmly pressing your thumbs over your scowl lines.

6. Form a "V" with the index and middle finger of each hand. Make 8 firm, upward strokes from the corners of the mouth to the tops of the ears, then start at the edge of the nostrils and repeat.

7. Extend the fingers of both hands and go over your entire face 5 times with small, circular motions. If you encounter any painful spots, pause and apply direct pressure for a few seconds to relieve tension and ease the discomfort.

8. Conclude the massage by tapping your fingers over your skin, beginning at the base of the throat and ending at the temple pressure points. Remove the lotion with tissues and a warm-water rinse.

In his late forties, George was still regarded as the "fair-haired young man" of his company, and maintaining this image was vital to his climb up the corporate ladder. When his wife began a regimen of before-bed facial massage and exercise, he decided to join her. Within two weeks George realized that his face-lifting endeavors had produced a bonus—his skin's increased smoothness and elasticity made shaving much easier!

Face-lifting exercises

Practiced persistently on a daily basis, exercise can restore lost strength to facial muscles and elasticity to their supporting tissues. Devise your own regimen from the following options, with or without an application of this stimulating cream applied to the jowl and under-chin area: 1 egg white, 1 tablespoon milk, 1 teaspoon each honey, liquid camphor, and mint extract; whisked to blend. Smooth on the mixture and let it dry. After completing your exercises, rinse with cool water and apply a moisturizer.

- Press the heels of your hands firmly against the crow's feet area, elevate your chin slightly, and open your mouth about an inch. Wrinkle your nose, contract your neck muscles, and smile as broadly as you can. Hold for 6 seconds. Relax and repeat 10 times.

- With your head thrown back, try to bite an imaginary apple. Relax and repeat 10 times.

- Open your mouth wide and try to contract your neck muscles at the same time. Repeat 10 times. Then open your mouth again and pull your lips in over your teeth. Pretend you are chewing by closing and opening your mouth 10 times.

- Stick out your chin and position your lower teeth over the upper ones. Nod your head up and down as you tun from far left to far right. Relax and repeat for a total of 10 left-to-right swings, then repeat the sequence from right-to-left.

- With your lips slightly parted, move your jaw from side to side as far as possible. Relax a few seconds between 10 repetitions. Then press your tongue against the roof of your mouth as forcefully as you can for a slow count of 6. Relax and repeat 3 times.

- Close your mouth but keep your teeth a quarter of an inch apart. Suck your cheeks between your teeth and hold for 6 seconds. Relax and repeat 3 times.

- Clench your back teeth, hold for 6 seconds, then release and drop your jaw. Slowly bring your jaw up again and bite down on your back molars for another 6 seconds. Relax and repeat for a total of 10 clenchings.

- Without lifting either shoulder, try to touch your left shoulder with your left ear and your right shoulder with your left ear. Repeat 3 times for each side. Follow this exercise by slowly circling your head 5 times to the right and 5 times to the left.

- Play turtle by pushing your neck out as far as it will go without moving your shoulders. Hold for 6 seconds, then slowly pull your chin in as far as you can toward your throat. Hold that position for 6 seconds, then relax and repeat several times.

- Wring a lightweight terry towel out of warm water, twist it into a rope and firmly but gently seesaw it under your chin with upward, outward motions.

- Lie on your back across a bed. With shoulders supported, let your head hang over the edge, then slowly raise and lower it 10 times.

- Squat with your buttocks resting on your heels, hands on your knees, and back straight. Thrust your hands out in front of you with fingers spread. Look up toward the ceiling with eyes wide open. Stick your tongue out and down as far as possible, then up to try to touch your nose. Hold this ungainly pose for a few moments; exhale deeply and relax. Repeat 5 times. (This Oriental yoga position, called "The Lion," tones muscles in both face and throat.)

Double-chin lift

European salons espouse this doubly potent method for disposing of double chins. You can achieve the same results, and save airfare to Paris, by contriving a strap from a strip of 3-inch-wide elastic bandage placed under your chin and tied at the top of your head. To duplicate the salons' secret solution: Dissolve 1/2 teaspoon epsom salt in 2 tablespoons hot water, stir in 1 tablespoon glycerin and 1 teaspoon 10-percent menthol solution. Store tightly covered.

Saturate gauze-covered cotton rectangles or eye pads in the liquid, tuck them between the elastic strap and your chin, and wear the contraption for an hour a day. If the solution irritates your skin, rinse it off and dilute the mixture with water. Use it as strong as bearable to stimulate circulation and help strengthen weakened muscles.

Pectin instant face-lift solution:

Cover your hair with a shower cap or towel turban; apply an egg-white masque from Chapter 5, or blend the following ingredients for a Pectin face-lift solution:

1/2 cup mineral water

1 tablespoon liquid pectin

1/2 teaspoon *each* alum and lemon juice

1/8 teaspoon vitamin C crystals

Smooth a thin layer over your face, then dip the gauze in the remaining pectin mixture. Wind the saturated gauze (use dry gauze if you have egg on your face) around your face and head by looping it under your chin, then making several slightly overlapping layers before tying the ends together on top of your head. The gauze should be tight enough to feel firmly comfortable. Leave the mummy-mask in place for 20 minutes while it stiffens to mold facial contours. Remove the gauze and rinse off the residue.

❧ 8 ❧

Bathing Beauty: The Luxurious Way to Cleanse & Beautify Your Body

Dry bathing, accomplished by rubbing the body with a coarsely textured mitt or friction glove, is a European favorite for removing surface debris and leaving skin looking like polished marble. Sponge baths suffice for invalids, or when no other facilities are available. Showering is a fast, efficient method of coping with body-cleaning chores. Tub bathing is a stress-relieving mini-vacation, the luxurious way to cleanse and beautify.

From ancient Roman baths accommodating 20,000 to California hot tubs with room for eight, sociable soaking has been part of almost every culture. Fourth-century aristocrats had their own private baths (as well as indoor latrines with stone troughs for free-flow of sewage into the streets). Cleanliness, however, has not always been regarded as virtuous. Early Christian saints considered dirtiness an insignia of holiness, philosophers' filthy beards were proof of their austere lifestyle. During the Middle Ages and well into the nineteenth-century, European society consisted of the unwashed working class who stank of sweat, and the equally unwashed nobility who reeked of cover-up scents. Our present-day penchant for odor-free cleanliness makes daily ablutions a required ritual.

How to Control Perspiration and Body Odor

Men sweat. Women perspire. Regardless of terminology, evaporation of this natural moisture is essential for dissipating excess body heat accumulated from metabolic processes, muscular exertion, and external sources. *Eccrine* sweat glands (widely distributed over the body) are stimulated by heat, physical activity, or nervous tension. The *apocrine* sweat glands do not develop until puberty, are activated by pain, sexual excitement or emotional stress, and are concentrated under the arms and around the genitals, with additional outlets on men's backs. Males perspire more profusely than females, although excessive perspiration may be caused by hormonal fluctuations, then wane as glandular activity decreases with age. Studies reported in *American Health* (July 1987) found that aging skin cells contract to partially close off sweat ducts; women between 52 and 62 perspire 30 percent less than younger women.

Normal perspiration is odorless when secreted; "body odor" is produced by bacteria growing and decomposing in the liquid. Only in our well-scrubbed society is this natural fragrance deemed unpleasant; it once was considered so sexually appealing that "love philters" filled with sweat were worn as aphrodisiacs. There is no firm evidence relating the aluminum in commercial deodorants and antiperspirants with the high aluminum levels found in patients with Alzheimer's disease, but for those who prefer Mother Nature's alternatives, there are many.

How dietary control can also control perspiration

What we ingest can affect the amount and the scent of our perspiration.

- Caffeine or other stimulants in coffee, tea, chocolate, soft drinks, or over-the-counter medications may be responsible for excess perspiration due to nervous tension.
- Garlic and other pungent seasonings can produce odiferous perspiration.
- Sage. Experimental studies in Germany show that drinking a cup of sage tea every day reduces excessive perspiration;[19] tomato juice blenderized with a handful of fresh sage leaves is even more effective.
- Vitamins and minerals. Dietary supplements of B-complex and magnesium often help reduce the amount of odor-forming perspiration, and a 30 to 50 milligram tablet of zinc each day can perform a dramatic odor-disappearing act.

- Water. Drinking enough water to dilute as well as replace the pints of liquid the body pours out through the skin each day helps diminish perspiration odor.

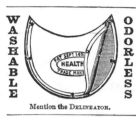
Dress shields have not changed appreciable since the 1890's; they still offer "protection against wetness."

Four natural deodorants and antiperspirants

Removing dead skin cells and existing bacteria by washing the armpits with a sudsy loofah during daily bathing usually forestalls odor problems. For additional freshness-security:

1. **Alcohol** is a deodorant and temporary antiperspirant. Apply rubbing alcohol, let dry, then dust with cornstarch.

2. **Baking soda and cornstarch.** Mix equal amounts of soda and cornstarch, or use cornstarch by itself—with a pinch of cloves, if desired. Apply to clean, dry armpits for a deodorant and mild antiperspirant.

3. **Clorophyll.** Chrysanthemum leaves, romaine or other leaf lettuce will produce a few drops of chlorophyll when the leaves are bruised and squeezed. Applied to the armpits, this liquid destroys odor-forming bacteria.

4. **Lavender oil.** Applying a single drop under each arm helps eliminate odor.

Six natural solutions for internal bathing

Advertisements notwithstanding, a certain degree of odor in the vaginal area is normal and, unless there is an infection or other physical dysfunction, daily douching is not only unnecessary but unwise.[149] When you do want a cleansing, refreshing douche, herbal infusions or other natural solutions are safer, and often more effective, than perfume-and-chemical-laden over-the-counter products.

- Aloe vera gel is noted for its healing properties. Mix 2 to 4 tablespoons with a quart of water.

- Baking soda. Dissolve 1 tablespoon in each quart of water.

- Garlic is helpful for yeast infections. Blender-puree 1 garlic clove with 1 cup water; strain, then add water to make 1 quart.

- Herbal combinations. For a cleansing-healing combo: Steep 1 teaspoon *each* horsetail and white oak bark in 1 cup boiling water. Strain, stir in 1 tablespoon aloe vera gel and 1/4 teaspoon garlic powder, and add 3 cups water.

   Make-ahead deodorant combo: Mix 1/2 cup each dried comfrey, myrtle, peppermint, and spearmint. Store in an airtight jar. When ready to use, bring 1/4 cup of the mixture to a boil in 2 cups water. Cover and steep for 15 minutes. Strain, then add 2 cups water.

- Individual herbal infusions. Prepare 2 cups regular strength tea from any of the following herbs: barberry, bistort (specific for vaginal bleeding), black walnut, blue cohosh, comfrey, fenugreek, ginger, golden seal, horsetail, marshmallow (specific for vaginal irritation), mint, myrrh, plantain, red raspberry, rose geranium, rosemary, slippery elm, uva ursi, white oak bark (specific for yeast infections), witch hazel bark. Strain through a fine sieve if not using tea bags, then combine with an equal amount of water before using as a douche.

- Vinegar. Add 1 tablespoon of either white or cider vinegar to 1 quart water, or use 2 tablespoons of any of the Cosmetic Vinegars described in Chapter 3.

Tub Time: Tips on Bathing in Bliss

Body cleansers vary from pure soaps (which leave a residue on both body and tub) to synthetic detergent-deodorant bars (which don't create any scum but may irritate sensitive skin). When tub bathing, the suggested procedure is to soak for 5 to 20 minutes, pull the plug, lather up and scrub while the water drains, then refill the tub with fresh water or turn on the shower to rinse. Loofahs slough off dead skin cells and long-handled brushes are handy for hard-to-reach areas. Men need to pay particular attention to the center of their backs where they have a high concentration of oil glands. To avoid the necessity for fresh-water rinsing, try one of these body-cleansing alternatives you can place in cotton bags or tie in cloth squares to use as scrubbers.

1/2 cup dry oatmeal

1/4 cup *each* cornmeal and powdered orris root

2 tablespoons *each* almond meal, cornmeal, and crushed elderflowers

Adding herbs, oils, or other enhancers turns bathing into a blissful interlude whether the purpose is to unwind tense nerves, relieve sore muscles (even the Spartans indulged in warm baths after athletic contests), soften and smooth rough or irritated skin, or simply refresh and invigorate. To transform a prosaic bathroom into your oasis of tranquility: dim the lights or turn them off and light a few candles, then tuck an inflatable bath pillow (or a rolled-up towel) under your head while you luxuriate.

Time and temperature: don't overdo

Water has an almost magical ability to either soothe or stimulate, depending on its temperature. A warm bath before bed summons the sandman, a 10 minute tepid soak followed by draining out half the water and refilling the tub with cool water energizes you for an evening engagement or for facing a new day. The vibrant beauty of hearty Scandinavians is not diminished by their practice of charging out of steamy saunas into snowbanks, but our health and beauty experts recommend no such extremes unless prescribed as medical treatment. Piping hot baths increase heart action and expand tiny capillaries into potential spider veins. Icy cold water constricts blood vessels and brutally jolts the nervous system. From comfortably warm to briskly cool is the temperature range most beneficial and beautifying. Although Benjamin Franklin reportedly read for hours while reclining in a tub he brought back from England, 15 to 20 minutes is considered sufficient wallowing time. Immersion for longer than 30 minutes can actually leech moisture from your skin, leaving it dry and uncomfortable.

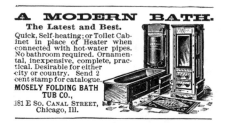

Prebath treatments for dry skin

- **Oil massage.** Stand in the empty tub. With deep, circular motions, coat yourself from neck to toe with cold-pressed vegetable or nut oil. Let it permeate for 2 to 3 minutes, then fill the tub and proceed with your bath.

- **Steam-heated treat.** Close the shower door or curtain and turn on the hot spray. While steam collects inside the shower, stand beside it on newspapers or an old towel and slather vegetable or nut oil over your face and body. Allow a few moments for it to penetrate before scraping off the excess with a rubber spatula or the back of a table knife. Turn off the water and stand in the closed shower until the steam dissipates, then fill the tub with warm water and soak for 10 to 20 minutes.

With Jeremy's promotion had come the opportunity for midday workouts, and the extra showers were taking their toll. Flaky patches, impervious to lotions, appeared all over his body and he came to the conclusion his skin was either washing off or wearing out. Hesitant about tub bathing (he visualized trying to wash while sitting in a few inches of water with his knees drawn up under his chin), Jeremy agreed to try this steam-heated combination only to save his skin. Which it did. And it was enjoyable. He actually looks forward to his relaxing Saturday-night bath but he can't resist the caustic comment: "You might know. . . I finally rate a key to the executive washroom, and now I have to stand on newspapers outside my own shower!"

Botanical Bathing: How to Enhance Your Bath with Herbs

Marie Antoinette, who bathed in a gilded tub, and Ninon de Lenclos, who scandalized seventeenth-century France with her entourage of avid male followers until she was in her eighties, attributed their beauty to herbal baths. Archaic directions for herbal bathing call for steeping the botanicals in boiling water for 20 minutes, then emptying solids as well as liquids into the bathwater. Today's plumbers might welcome service calls for herb-clogged drains, but emerging from a tub with a coating of soggy seeds and leaves has little appeal. For problem-free botanical bathing:

- Toss a dozen tea bags in the empty tub, run an inch or so of steamy hot water over them, then wait 10 minutes before filling the tub and joining the tea bags.
- Steep a minimum of 1/2 cup (ideally, 10 ounces) dried herbs in boiling water for 20 minutes. Strain. Pour the liquid in the tub, then spread the solids on a washcloth for a facial pack or use them as a cloth-encased scrubber. One young man, who is into herbs but not into tub bathing, scrubs with the herb-

filledwashcloth,thenusesthestrainedliquidasanafter-shower rinse.

- Fill a drawstring cloth bag with the herbs; or place them in the center of a square of doubled cheesecloth, pull up the corners and secure the bag with string, rubber bands, or grocery-store twisters. Hang this pouch over the tub spout waterfall as the tub fills; or, place the bag in a few inches of very hot water in the bottom of the tub for 10 minutes, then fill the tub and soak and scrub with the bagged botanicals. If neither you nor your favorite fellow have time for boiling water before bathing, simply anchor the giant tea bag to the shower spout for an herbal waterfall, then detach it for a final rubdown.

25 herbs and their unique benefits

For voluptuously velvety skin, swish a teaspoon of avocado oil in your bath after the herbs have been added, or include half a cup of miller's bran in your herbal bath. You can steep and strain the bran right along with the botanicals; or bag it separately or with your choice of herbs.

- **Bergamot** is used for relaxing and inducing sleep.
- **Blackberry leaves,** dried, crumbled, steeped and strained, invigorate the body and relieve sore muscles.
- **Camomile** is a comforting herb; soothing and relaxing, it has an anti-inflammatory effect on muscles.
- **Cloves** should be used sparingly, too much can numb the skin.
- **Comfrey,** used once or twice weekly, rejuvenates the skin.
- **Elderflowers** are mildly astringent and stimulating.
- **Eucalyptus leaves** make a body-stimulating bath especially enjoyed by the masculine contingent.
- **Ginger** is another bath pleaser; adding 1/4 cup of powdered ginger will chase a wintry chill and help rid the body of toxins. For a mid-summer zinger with male appeal, grate a large ginger root into boiling water and let it steep for 20 minutes. Strain the liquid into a tubful of tepid water, then wrap the solids for a spice-sponge to rev up circulation.
- **Hops,** basically a beer ingredient, calms the nerves to prepare you for sleep.
- **Jasmine** can be used for tropical scent plus skin smoothing.
- **Juniper berries,** the secret ingredient in gin, relieve pain and stimulate circulation to promote a rosy glow. (Adding a few

drops of juniper oil is said to have the same effect as 1/2 cup of the dried, crushed berries.)

- **Lavender** is used for fragrance, relaxation, and a clear complexion.
- **Mint** provides mental as well as physical soothing.
- **Mustard** soothes sore, tired muscles. Place 1 teaspoon dry mustard in a tub of water.
- **Oat straw** (the herb) has such a calming effect it is used as a remedy for insomnia.
- **Orange blossoms and leaves** have both been favorites for all-over skin beautifying since ancient Roman times.
- **Peppermint** is a tonic for oily or irritated skin, a before-bed nerve calmer, and a terrific cooler for hot days.
- **Pine needles** relieve nervous tension, especially if you fantasize about bathing in a peaceful primeval forest.
- **Plantain leaves** have healing properties. Steep the dried, crumbled leaves in boiling water, strain the liquid into your bath, then apply the solids to ailing skin.
- **Raspberry leaves** are astringently cleansing and refreshing.
- **Rosemary** soothes skin and regenerates the nervous system.
- **Sage,** when taken internally as a tea, aids mental alertness; as a bath additive it is a sleep inducer.
- **Thyme and valerian** are soporifics, great for "unwinding" at any time of day or night.
- **Yarrow** inhibits infections and is recommended for oily or blemished skin.
- **Yellow dock** relieves itchy skin. Steep and strain before adding to the tub.

You can individualize your beauty bath by blending two or more of the following aromatic herbs: acacia, angelica root, cinnamon, cloves (no more than 1 teaspoon per tub), lavender, lemon peel, lovage root, marigold, myrtle leaves, orange leaves, pennyroyal, rose geranium, rosemary, sandalwood, verbena.

Six advantages of using dried herb mixtures in your bath

Specific combinations of dried herbs are especially effective for:

- **Deep cleansing.** Steep 2 or 3 tablespoons *each* hibiscus, lemon grass, peppermint, rosemary, witch hazel leaves or bark in boiling water. Strain. Add the liquid to your bath, wrap the solids in a washcloth to use as a scrubber.

- **Dry, itchy skin.** (See also the sunburn-relieving baths in Chapter 9.) Prepare equal amounts of camomile, fennel, lovage, peppermint, rosemary, sage, and yarrow by any one of the herbal-bath methods.

  Or, mix 1/4 cup *each* almond meal, cornmeal, oatmeal, and orris root. Secure the mixture in a cloth bag or washcloth; squeeze out the milkiness while you are soaking, then rub your skin with the bag.

- **Rejuvenating and energizing.** Mix equal parts of alfalfa, comfrey, orange peel, and parsley; or of basil, bay leaves, fennel, and mint (a masculine favorite); or of lavender, orange blossoms, and rose petals; or of juniper, lavender or rosemary, and rose geranium. Or, combine 3/4 cup jasmine with 1/4 cup orange blossoms.

- **Relaxing.** Mix equal amounts of camomile, horsetail, rosemary, pine needles, and valerian; or of camomile, peppermint, and rosemary; or of comfrey, lavender, mint, and rosemary (with thyme added if desired); or of comfrey, marigold, and yarrow.

- **Relieving stiff muscles.** For best results, massage the sore muscles while you are soaking with strawberry leaves and sage, mixed half-and-half; or with equal amounts of agrimony, camomile, and mugwort.

- **Spicy luxuriating.** For a Parisian extravaganza, steep 2 tablespoons *each* bay leaves, lavender, marjoram, rosemary, and thyme in 2 cups of boiling water for 15 minutes. Strain and add to your bath with 1/2 cup cognac.

Nine Natural Additives for Pampering Your Skin While You Bathe

1. **Glycerin** silkens your skin while it prevents "ring around the tub." Swish a tablespoonful into the water; add rose water for fragrance, if desired.

Cucumber glycerin: For a skin-rejuvenating treatment, simmer an unpeeled, sliced cucumber in unsalted water until tender. Strain off the solids and add the liquid to your bath with 2 tablespoons of glycerin.

2. **Honey.** Add 1 tablespoon to your tub to soften your skin.

3. **Lemon.** To reduce the oils on your skin, and to unjangle your nerves, swirl a cup of fresh lemon juice in the bathwater.

4. **Milk.** The words "milk bath" evoke a vision of Cleopatra lolling seductively in her swan-shaped tub, surrounded by a procession of Nubian slaves decanting ornate jeroboams of camel's milk. Between that exotic scene and the simplicity of swishing a cup of powdered milk into the tub as it fills, lie 2,000 years of experience with its skin-softening, soothing benefits. The recent revival of interest in milk bathing has led several cosmetic companies to include packets of scented "milk" in their lines, but the predominance of preservatives and chemicals in commercial products makes their virtue questionable. Mother Nature still knows best. Whether fluid or dry, whole or skim, just-plain-milk added to your bathwater produces the sensation of floating in a soft, warm cloud—without leaving a sticky residue.

Two to three cups of fluid milk, or one cup of instant dry milk (noninstant powdered milk turns into lumpy globs if not first dissolved in water or encased in a cloth bag) will soften hard water, smooth and firm your skin. For even more spectacular results, indulge in one of these combos.

Oil and milk pamper your skin and dispense with dry flakies. Reverse the usual procedure by cleansing before entering your beauty bath—milk and oil may mix with water, but soap gets scummy—and be cautious when exiting from any bath containing oil, as both you and the tub will be slippery. Depending upon how dry you are, add 1/2 teaspoon to 1/2 cup almond, avocado, wheat germ, or other unsaturated oil and 2 to 6 cups fluid milk (or the equivalent in instant dry milk) to the tub as it fills. Swish to combine, then luxuriate for at least 15 minutes before polishing off dead skin with a loofah or bath brush.

Salty milk is a potent solution for transforming rough, scaly skin into silky smoothness. Dissolve 1 cup of table salt in a pan of boiling water. Pour it into your tub and mix in 4 cups of instant nonfat dry milk (or 3 quarts of fluid milk). Soak, then scrub with a washcloth or loofah.

Simulated milk bath: To reap the skin-smoothing benefits of a genuine milk bath, stir 1 cup cornstarch with mineral oil to make a thick liquid; mix into the water as the tub fills.

Super-soother for skin-pampering nourishing: simmer 1/2 cup barley in a quart of water until tender. Place 1/4 cup *each* almond meal, oatmeal, and orris root (if available) in a cloth bag or a square of doubled cheesecloth and fasten securely. Strain the barley liquid into the bathtub as it fills. Add the filled cloth bag and 1 cup instant dry milk. As you soak, gently rub your skin with the squishy bag.

Tea with milk and honey makes a milk bath good enough to drink. Mix 2 cups double-strength camomile tea with 1/2 cup honey. Stir into your bathwater with 4 cups instant dry milk (or 3 quarts fluid milk).

5. Oatmeal with bran and bay leaves are perfect post-sports bath enhancers. Combine 1/4 cup *each* dry oatmeal and miller's bran with 2 tablespoons crushed bay leaves; simmer for an hour in 2 quarts of water before straining the liquid into the tub. For a more femininely scented version, substitute 2 tablespoons of lavender for the bay leaves.

6. Oils. Olive and sesame oils were the ancient Roman and Egyptian favorites; tropical-island inhabitants utilized coconut oils. Here's how to manufacture your own coconut oil:

Drain and reserve the milk from 2 coconuts. Grate the meat, add 1/2 cup of the coconut milk, and squeeze the mixture through your fingers for several minutes. Strain into a nonmetal cooking container and simmer the liquid for an hour. Strain again and bottle. If you are a perfectionist, you can clarify the oil by adding 3 times as much water as you have oil, boiling the mixture for 15 minutes, pouring it into a glass bowl, and cooling it until you can skim off the clarified product before discarding the water.

Bathing in an emulsion of oil and water helps restore the moisture lost through the assaults of detergents, counteracts chemical dyes from clothing, repairs skin damage from exposure to heat and cold, and relieves dry, itchy skin. The soft film of oil clings, even after toweling, to leave you sleek and smooth. Any vegetable or nut oil produces equally beautifying results when one-fourth teaspoon to one-fourth cup is swirled in the water. For fragrant silkiness, you can dilute the homemade Attar of Roses from Chapter 3 with almond or olive oil.

Almond bath oil. Emulsify 1 cup almond oil and 1 tablespoon detergent shampoo with an electric blender or a rotary egg beater. (Include 1/2 teaspoon of your favorite perfume, if desired.) Bottle and shake well before pouring 2 tablespoons into your tub. The shampoo breaks the oil into fine globules, making it cling to all seven million of your pores.

Apricot bath soak

2 tablespoons wheat germ oil

1 tablespoon melted butter

3 large, ripe apricots

1 cup whole milk, divided

2 small eggs or 1 extra large egg

1/4 cup yogurt

2 tablespoons witch hazel

1 teaspoon apple cider vinegar

Combine the wheat germ oil and butter. Let stand while liquefying the pitted apricots with 1/2 cup of the milk. Strain. Return the liquid to the blender, add all other ingredients and whir until emulsified. Use 1/3 of the mixture for a luxurious, skin nourishing bath. Store the remainder in the refrigerator.

Floral bath oil. The Charitable Physitian, written in 1639 by Philbert Guibert Esq. & Physitian Regent in Paris, recommends the "enfleurage" method of procuring rose oil:

To Make Oyle of Roses

Take a pound of red Rose buds, beat them in a marble morter with a wooden pestle, then put them into an earathen pot, and pour upon them four pound of oyle of olives, letting them infuse the space of a month in the Sunne, or in the chimney corner, stirring of them sometimes, then heat it, and press it and strain it, and put it into the same pot or other vessel to keep.

Dr. Guibert's method must have been effective and might apply to producing other floral oils, but there is a less time-consuming way to transform a bottle of salad oil into an exotic bath enhancer.

For your floral oil you will need a 9-by-12-by-2-inch glass pan; a roll of absorbent cotton; clear glass to cover the pan; a pint of oil; tincture of benzoin; and gardenia, heliotrope, honeysuckle, jasmine, magnolia, rose, stock, verbena, violet, water lily, or other scented flower petals.

Place a layer of cotton in the bottom of the pan. blend 1 teaspoon benzoin with 2 cups almond or other natural oil; drizzle 1/2 cup of it over the cotton. Arrange a thick layer of unsprayed, dust free flower petals over the oil-saturated cotton, cover with another layer of cotton, and pour in the remaining oil. Top with clear glass and place near a sunny window. Once each day, for at least three days, lift the top layer of cotton, remove the old flowers, and replace with fresh petals. When the scent reaches the desired strength, squeeze the oil out of the cotton, strain out the flower petals, and funnel your perfumed oil into a lightproof, airtight bottle.

7. **Salts.** As sold commercially, "bath salts" are water softeners. To manufacture your own: Place 2 cups borax in a jar. Stir in 1/4 teaspoon of your favorite perfume. Cover and let stand 24 hours. Stir in another 1/4 teaspoon perfume and store tightly closed. Use 2 or 3 tablespoons for each bath.

Epsom salt has a reviving effect on the body when 1/2 cup is added to the bathwater. A solution of 1 pound per tub is a restorative for overworked muscles and ligaments if you alternate underwater massaging with relaxing.

Sea salt (or table salt mixed half-and-half with epsom salt) also has a beneficial effect on sore muscles, cleanses pores, and revs up weary bodies. Use 1 or 2 cups for each bath.

Sea salt scrub is an allover exfoliant to depose dead skin cells and restore rough skin to seductive smoothness. Mix 1 cup sea salt with enough water, milk, or oil to form a paste. Stand in a partially filled tub while vigorously rubbing the salt mixture over your wet body. Fill the tub with warm water, then soak and bathe as usual.

Table salt is said to help guard against vaginal infections when 1/2 cup is dissolved in the bathwater.[128]

8. **Vinegar** can help relieve achy muscles or flaky, itchy skin. It will both relax and invigorate your body when 1 cup is added to your bath. For pizzazz plus fragrance, use one of the cosmetic vinegars from Chapter 3.

9. **Wheat flour** doesn't sound glamorous, but when it is encased in a muslin bag, or heaped on an old handkerchief and tied into a packet, it is a wonderful skin softener. Hang your bag or packet over the spout as the tub fills, then remove it to gently massage your body as you soak.

For dry skin, put 2 tablespoons *each* whole wheat flour and powdered milk in the bag.

For oily or blemished skin, use 2 tablespoons *each* whole wheat flour, camomile, and lemon balm.

Enticing After-bath Moisturizers

To seal in your skin's newly acquired moisture (the January 1988 issue of *Health* reports that a 20-minute soak creates temporary skin hydration of up to 40 percent), smooth on one of the facial moisturizers from Chapter 4, petroleum jelly, your own floral bath oil, or either of these harem-favorite lotions.

MOROCCO MOISTURIZER: Combine 1/4 cup *each* almond oil, honey, and strained, fresh lemon juice in the top of a double boiler or small saucepan. Heat and stir until thoroughly blended. Bottle and refrigerate.

SULTAN'S SECRET: Pulverize a handful of sesame seeds in an electric blender. Continue blending while gradually adding water until you have a milky lotion. Strain and store in the refrigerator.

How to Make Your Own Natural Bath Powder

Commercial dusting powders and talcs may contain chemical additives or perfumes that irritate sensitive skin and can cause allergic reactions or internal damage.[32] For the delight without the danger, try these natural options:

Arrowroot, cornstarch, or old-fashioned laundry starch are perfume-free and as absorbant as talcum powder.

Fuller's earth is a harmless, basic-beige dusting powder.

Rice flour, sifted until fluffy, was a preferred powder for bodies as well as faces until twentieth-century cosmetology became a profitable industry.

Scented powders

- **Gardenia.** If you harbor fond memories of your senior prom, and have access to a gardenia bush, fill a pint container with fresh gardenias, add as much cornstarch (or other talc substitute) as possible, and cover tightly. Shake the mixture each 8 hours and replace the gardenias every other day until the powder is as fragrant as desired.

- **Herbal dusting powders** require either a mortar and pestle or a spice-coffee grinder to pulverize the dried botanicals before combining with any of the talc substitutes.

  Floral: Mix equal amounts of powdered lavender, orris root, and rose petals. Stir in cornstarch to double the total quantity.

  Spicy: Blend equal parts of powdered cloves and sage. Match their combined amount with orris root, then stir in arrowroot to double the volume.

  Springtime essence: Combine equal amounts of powdered lilac blossoms, orris root, and violet blooms. Add cornstarch to triple their total volume.

How to Make Splash-On Cologne

In a glass jar, combine 1 pint ethyl alcohol or 80 proof vodka; 2 teaspoons oil of lavender; and 1 teaspoon *each* oil of balm, oil of lemon, oil of orange, and oil of rosemary. Keep tightly covered and shake three times a day for one week. Strain through moistened coffee-filter paper into an attractive bottle with an airtight stopper.

❧ 9 ❧

Sun Smarts:
How to Have Fun
Without the Burn

The ancients paid homage to the sun as a god but only during this century have sun worshippers prostrated themselves beneath its rays to darken their skins. "Sun bronzed" replaced "alabaster white" as a status symbol when laborers moved indoors from fields to factories, and the discovery that sunshine is the primary source of vitamin D encouraged sun exposure. According to the March 1988 issue of *Men's Health*, sunlight is sexually stimulating and may improve the odds of child conception by increasing ovulation in women and sperm production in men. Along with appreciation of its benefits, however, has come awareness of sunlight's potential dangers.

How to Avoid the Hazards of Sunning

Frequent misting with water is no longer advised as a tanning aid. The water cools your skin as it evaporates, enabling you to prolong your sunning without discomfort, but it increases the potential for skin damage. As explained in Health (January 1988), skin cells flatten out when they are wet and allow more of the burning rays to permeate. Sun damage accumulates slowly, often requiring years to overpower the body's natural defenses. This cumulative overexposure is now being held responsible for premature aging of the skin, most skin cancers, and many cataracts.

Photoaging

Differing from normal aging, *photoaging* results from ultraviolet rays penetrating the epidermis, dilating dermal blood vessels, and clumping the elastin and collagen which support the skin—thus creating skin sags and wrinkles, plus other problems such as:

- *Liver spots/age spots.* Byproducts of photoaging, not liver dysfunction, these small, flat, liver-colored spots on the skin are medically identified as *senile lentigines* (from the Latin "old" and "brown spots") because of the years of accumulated sun exposure required to produce them.
- *Droopy noses.* In the December 1987 issue of *Prevention,* Dr. Albert N. Kligman states that noses react to sunlight with more than temporary redness; long term exposure can damage the cartilage and make the tip of your nose droop.

Photosensitivity

Interaction between the sun's ultraviolet rays and cosmetic ingredients, drugs, or foods may cause brown splotches, an itchy rash, or other unpleasantries. Shaving immediately before sun exposure magnifies the sensitivity of male faces or female legs.

- Colognes, perfumes, and after-shave lotions may leave semi-permanent brown spots on your skin if you apply them before going out in the sun.
- Deodorants and deodorant soaps containing hexachlorophene can bring out an itchy, red rash if used before sunbathing.
- Drugs and medications, such as tetracycline and other antibiotics, diuretics, and tranquilizers can make you especially prone to sunburn. Oral contraceptives cause some women to develop a *pregnancy mask* (a pattern of dark blotches around the eyes) from exposure to the sun.
- Foods that can be photosensitizing include celery, citrus fruits, figs, parsnips, and vanilla.

Cataracts and skin cancer

Even more disturbing than rashes, blotches, or premature wrinkles nis the possibility of eye damage or skin melanoma. Studies have demonstrated that excessive exposure to the sun results in cloudy vision with increased incidence of cataract,[129] and the *University of California, Berkeley Wellness Letter* (June 1988) reports that approximately one-tenth of the million cataracts removed each year in the United States are sun related.

Statistics given in the *Journal of the American Academy of Dermatology* (December 1987 issue) show that between the years 1980 and 1987 new melanomas in the United States increased 83 percent, while the population rose by only 10.6 percent. Doctors and researchers attribute these skin cancers to cumulative effects from the sun-worshipping 1960s and 1970s because of the 15 to 20 years required for melanomas to develop; and, as reported in the October 1987 issue of *Trends*, it is estimated that at least one out of every seven Americans eventually will have one or more skin cancers.

Tanning Without the Sun

Bronzing gels for sunless tans are presumed harmless but are still undergoing safety tests. Tanning salons are touted as being safer than the sun because their high-intensity light sources emit fewer of the burning UVB rays. However, according to reports in *Health* (June 1987) and *University of California, Berkeley Wellness Letter* (February 1989), man-made ultraviolet rays are from 5 to 100 times more powerful than those of the midday sun, penetrate the skin more deeply, and are proportionately more likely to cause premature aging or melanomas. The American Academy of Dermatology has requested that health warnings be mandated in tanning parlors as they are on cigarette packages.

If you can't deal directly with the sun, you might try this natural skin bronzer with astringent properties that offer a beautifying bonus of pore refining and skin tightening: Brew strong black pekoe tea by steeping 3 tea bags in 1 cup boiling water until comfortably warm. Stand in the bathtub and sponge the tea over your face and body with the tea bags. Let the liquid dry for a few minutes, then blot (do not rub) with a soft towel. Repeat daily until as dark as desired, then twice a week for maintenance.

Playing Safe in the Sunshine

Lurking indoors during daylight hours is not the only option. You can apply a sunscreen, wear sunglasses, and, for prolonged exposure while working or playing in the sun, a hat with a brim wide enough to shade your nose. To test your clothing for sun safety, hold the garment up to a light. Loosely woven fabrics offer scant protection, tightly woven cloth such as blue denim is excellent.

Sunscreens

Sunscreens absorb, reflect, or scatter the ultraviolet radiation that causes sunburn, yet permit some of the less-dangerous, tanning rays to travel through to the skin. Moisturizing substances are incorporated to replace tanning lotions and help prevent an aftermath of flaky dryness. They are rated from 2 to 35 according to their SPF (sun protection factor), with 2 providing twice the natural skin protection, and 35 presenting an almost impenetrable barrier under laboratory conditions, but diffusion by perspiration or swimming can reduce their potency. The official recommendation is to apply the sunscreen 15 minutes before going outside and reapply it several times during sunbathing.[25] This consistent protection allows your skin to begin repairing existing photoaging damage by building a new network of collagen, connective tissue, and elastin fibers.[26] For tanning with a sunscreen:

If you are in a hurry to obtain a tan, and do not burn easily, use SPF 4.

If you tan normally, start with SPF 15, then reduce to SPF 10 after establishing a base tan.

If you burn easily, use SPF 15 to 35 and do not overindulge in sunbathing.

Sunglasses

Eyes, too, need protection from the sun. Eyelids are subject to skin cancer, and, in addition to the increased potential for cataracts, unprotected eyes lose 50 percent of their night vision after a day at the beach or on the ski slopes; it may be a week before your eyes recover from a two-week holiday in the sun.

Eskimos wear gogglelike pieces of bone carved with narrow slits to shield their eyes, and Nero watched the Christians versus lions arena-entertainments through an emerald lens. However, neither shields nor color can provide the protection our eyes need; they require specially ground lenses to filter out the rays that damage eyes and the tender skin surrounding them. When you shop for sunglasses, make sure they are designated "Z-80.3" or have an SPF rating of 15. For protection against sun reflection from water or snow, experts advise opaque side pieces on the glasses.

Tips for protecting extra-sensitive areas

Eyes, ears, nose, and throat. These are especially sensitive thin-skinned areas. While your sunscreen-lotioned body is soaking up direct sunlight, covering your eyes with gauze pads dunked in cool water, pekoe or slippery-elm tea can prevent puffy-eyed evenings and future wrinkles. If you remain in the sun very long, your ears, too, may need the protection of cotton pads. A plastic nose cover can keep you from looking like W. C. Fields, and extra slatherings of sunscreen should avoid the possibility of becoming a "red neck."

Hair, natural or tinted, may redden or blanch from exposure to the sun's rays; permed hair can be further weakened. The combination of sun and perspiration, especially when compounded with ocean salt or swimming-pool chlorine, can be disastrously destructive. For shiny, manageable hair—instead of a headful of discolored, strawlike strands—comb in a bit of conditioner; cover your head with a scarf, terrycloth turban, or hat while sunning; wear a bathing cap when swimming; and rinse or shampoo your hair after each exposure.

Hands and feet deserve their fair share of attention and lotion; sun-blistered feet and blotchy, sun-puffed hands can spoil the effect of an otherwise perfect tan.

Thirst Quenchers: What to drink while sunning

Replenishing the fluid your body loses through perspiration is essential. What to drink while sunning? Water, lemonade, and diluted fruit juices are ideal choices. If you feel faint or nauseous, stir 1/4 teaspoon baking soda and 1/8 teaspoon salt into a glass of lemonade or water, then sip about half of it. The salt and soda provide quick replacement of critical minerals lost in the perspiration. If your internal unease lingers, drink the rest of the mixture.

- Alcoholic beverages are mild diuretics that deplete the body of water and make you more thirsty. They also constrict blood vessels (making you feel hotter) and rob you of B vitamins required for the tanning process...saving them for the shade is suggested.

- Caffeine increases skin sensitivity and the chances of burning before tanning, so caffeine-containing coffee, tea, and soft drinks are not recommended while sunning.

How to Cultivate a Healthy Tan

Suntanning is a complex process. Pigment cells in the skin undergo an immediate biochemical change that darkens them within a few hours. Exposure to ultraviolet rays also triggers a delayed reaction which stimulates the production of more pigment cells, and continues to deepen the tan for up to 96 hours.

You can acquire a light tan just by watching the sun worshipers. Fifty percent of the sun's tanning rays bounce off pavement, pool decks, sand, and water to reach you under a beach umbrella, boat canopy, or shaded lanai; and they penetrate lightweight clothing. Spectacular tans must be carefully cultivated. Your geographical location, chronological age, and how brown you want to be determines the best way to go about achieving your goal.

- If you're tanning while traveling, it's wise to bear in mind that the sun's rays are more intense in equatorial regions and at high altitudes than they are in your own backyard.
- The body's metabolic balance changes with age; your tolerance for sunshine may be much less when you are 50 than it was when you were 15.
- Clouds can't be counted on; approximately 80 percent of the sun's burning rays seep through smoggy cloud cover.

Dark-haired Lorna had no trepidation about sunbathing. She had tanned beautifully in the high-altitude Colorado Rockies and on the Arizona desert—and she never burned. The vacation day she scheduled for California sunbathing, however, proved to be a disastrous learning experience. The sky was overcast, the fog didn't roll out, the smog didn't lift, and an almost chilling breeze blew across the sand. Disappointed, Lorna read the book she had brought along, and waited for the sun to appear. It didn't. But prickling, burning sensations commenced on the drive back to the hotel. Lorna subdued the discomfort of her beet-red skin with cool baths and vitamin-E oil . . . but well remembers the burn-with-blisters resulting from a sunless day at the beach.

How to time your tanning

The sun's rays are the most powerful when directly overhead; less penetrating in the early morning and late afternoon. Besides adhering to the old dictum of "not between 10 a.m. and 2 p.m.," you can take advantage of modern technology to monitor your tanning time. There are solar-powered meters that give a digital readout of the ultraviolet level, and adhesive strips that change color according to your level of sun exposure. Watching your watch is a less expensive alternative.

Starting with two brief sunning sessions a day is the recommended approach. Blondes and redheads with fair skin and blue eyes have little defense against the sun. Their beginning exposure time should be limited to no more than 20 minutes. Brunettes with darker, less sensitive skin have more natural protection, and may be able to double that time. Deep olive to black skin provides a built-in sun shield against burning but is not immune to the hazards of sun-induced skin cancer and aging.[150]

As your tan develops, your skin thickens and you can gradually lengthen your time in the sun. The moment you notice signs of redness, feel nauseous, or have cold, clammy skin, however, go indoors to avoid a sunburn or the possibility of sunstroke.

Enhancing your tan with natural lotions

To pamper your skin and enhance the golden glow acquired with sunscreen protection, slather on any of the natural substances once used as tanning lotions.

- Aloe vera gel or petroleum jelly.
- Vegetable oils, singly or in combinations such as avocado or almond oil mixed with wheat germ oil.
- Cocoa-butter cream made by blending 1/4 cup coconut oil with 1/4 cup melted cocoa butter.
- Yogurt cream, prepared by placing the following ingredients in a blender container and whirring them until smooth:

> 3 tablespoons water-dispersible lecithin
> 2 tablespoons yogurt
> 2 tablespoons *each* avocado oil and sesame oil
> 1 tablespoon water
> 1 teaspoon potato flour

- Tea lotion, an old favorite that can be stored in the refrigerator for up to three months.

  1/2 cup water
  4 tea bags of regular pekoe tea
  3/4 cup wheat germ oil
  1/2 cup sesame oil
  1/4 cup apple cider vinegar
  1 teaspoon iodine

Bring the water to a boil, add the tea bags, cover and let steep until room temperature. Whisk the oils with the vinegar, then beat in the tea and the remaining ingredients.

Tanning supplements

- *Vitamin A*: Studies indicate that additional vitamin A plus a bone-meal supplement increases the protection provided by sunscreens.[130] A daily capsule of 25,000 units of beta carotene (which the body converts to vitamin A as needed) helps reduce night blindness resulting from exposure to bright light.
- *B Complex*: B vitamins are necessary for the production of tanning pigments, so your body may rob its stores to pay for your bronzed beauty, or you may burn instead of tan. Eating more B-vitamin-containing foods (see Vitamin and Mineral Chart) and/or taking a B-complex supplement helps your system assist the sun.

  According to nutritionist Adelle Davis, persons who sunburn readily and those who are susceptible to skin cancers have unusually high B-vitamin requirements and can increase their sun-tolerance by taking 1,000 milligrams of PABA plus a 30-milligram tablet of zinc daily.[48, 49]
- *Vitamin C*: A lack of this vitamin may be responsible for a spotty tan. Eating vitamin-C-rich foods (see Vitamin and Mineral Chart) and taking supplemental C also strengthens skin tissues to help prevent photoaging.

What to Do When You're Overdone:
Tips on Relieving Sunburn Pain

Overexposure to the sun causes tiny blood vessels in the dermis to dilate. Within a few hours blood serum from these dilated vessels seeps into skin tissues and distends the surface. Blisters erupt from a severe sunburn and, eventually, the top layer of skin peels off. Besides the temporary discomfort, repeated sunburns can instigate an assortment of skin problems. As reported in *Prevention* (May 1988), blistering sunburns double the chances of developing skin cancer. Skin may become leathery, the underlying tissue lose its elasticity (a degenerative change called *solar elastosis*), and wrinkles form. Tiny red spots from burst capillaries may appear on fair skins; spider or splotchy veins may worsen from being expanded by the heat; and existing freckles and little brown blotches become more obvious.

Underestimating the power of the sun is what usually leads to a sunburn. Overcast skies present no barrier to its burning rays, and neither does water. In addition to allowing penetration by ultraviolet rays, water acts as a prism to concentrate the sun's heat—in the same way that a magnifying glass can be used to start a fire with solar power.

How to Relieve Sunburn Pain

Hardy souls may swear by a hot shower to extinguish sunburn fire, turn the red into tan, and prevent blistering, but most of us prefer gentle cooling as the first step. The force of water from a shower can be painful; soaking your sizzling body for 15 minutes in a tub of cool water eases the burning and replaces some of the moisture in your dehydrated skin. While you lie there soaking and vowing never again to overexpose, placing moist tea bags or thin slices of raw potato or cucumber over your sun-puffed eyelids helps reduce their swelling. Adding one of these naturally soothing and healing substances to your bath will make the total relief more immediate, and more long lasting.

- Swish 2 cups of apple cider vinegar, or 2 cups of fluid milk, or 2/3 cup of instant nonfat dry milk in the bathwater. To further pamper your mistreated skin, add a tablespoon of almond oil.

- Place 2 cups of cornstarch in the tub; mix with the water while the tub fills.

- "Old-tyme receipts" say to place 1 cup of oatmeal in a drawstring bag or a muslin diaper with the corners tied together. If you don't happen to have either item, encase the oatmeal in doubled cheesecloth or in a nylon knee-hi. Let the container soak with you in the tub, then squeeze it to drizzle the oatmeal juices over your skin. If sharing your bath with a cup of uncooked porridge in a snagged stocking offends your sensibilities, simply swish in

1/2 cup of *colloidal oatmeal* (a commercially available mixture of powdered oatmeal, lanolin, and mineral oil).

- Place 2 ounces of dried rosemary in 2 cups of water and bring to a boil. Cover and let steep for 30 minutes. Strain, then pour into the filling tub. To save time, substitute rosemary tea bags: let the water run until steamy, put the plug in the tub and toss in a handful of the tea bags. Shut off the water as soon as the bags are covered, let them "steep" for 10 minutes, then fill the tub with tepid water and join the floating tea bags.

Dousing or compressing

If a tub bath is not feasible, you can cool your sun-abused skin with any of these liquids—sprayed, splashed, or smoothed on, or made into cloth compresses.

- *Alcohol.* Add 1 tablespoon rubbing alcohol to 2 cups cold water.
- *Almond milk.* In an electric blender, whir 1 cup water with 1/4 cup almond meal. Strain before applying.
- *Alum.* Dissolve 1 teaspoon alum in 2 cups of water.
- *Apple cider vinegar.* It doesn't smell any better than it ever did, and you may have to repeat the application every 20 minutes, but splashing on vinegar does bring relief, just as it did hundreds of years ago.
- *Baking soda.* Dissolve 3 tablespoons soda in 1 quart cold water.
- *Milk.* Saturate cloths with cold milk and apply to the burned areas.
- *PABA lotion.* Dissolve 1 teaspoon crushed PABA tablets in 1/4 cup water. Sponge over burned areas.
- *Pekoe tea or sage tea.* Make a strong infusion from 4 tea bags in 1 cup of boiling water. Add ice cubes to cool, then pat the liquid over your skin with the moist tea bags.
- *Potato juice.* Liquefy raw potatoes in an electric juicer or blender, then douse your skin to help remove the heat and relieve the pain.

Pain-halting coatings for your skin

After the initial cooling, coat your sunburned areas with one of these air-excluding substances because, as Dr. Chase explains in his 1904 book of home cures,[67] the oxygen in the air coming in contact with the skin is what produces sensations of smarting and burning.

- *Aloe vera gel*. This ancient remedy for burns is cooling, soothing (one of its constituents is a chemical cousin of aspirin), and healing.
- *Baking soda or equal parts of baking soda and cornstarch*. Blend with water or milk to make a paste. Cover the burned areas and do not rinse off for an hour.
- *Cream or yogurt*. Apply over the burned areas. Leave on until dry, then rinse off and reapply to reap all of the pain-relieving, healing benefits.
- *Cucumber*. Puree a chopped cucumber in an electric blender with 1 tablespoon witch hazel and 1 teaspoon honey. Pat over your sunburn and leave on for 15 minutes before rinsing off.
- *Egg yolk*. Folk healers advise smearing raw egg yolk over sunburned areas and letting it dry for 30 minutes before washing off.
- *Honey*. Plain honey is recognized as one of the best ointments for burns. Mixing it half-and-half with wheat germ oil incorporates the healing benefits of vitamin E. For severely burned areas, try whirring honey and wheat germ oil in a blender with dry comfrey tea to make a thick paste.
- *Laundry starch*. Old-fashioned laundry starch, prepared as for starching shirt collars, brings radical relief to sunburned skin.
- *Mayonnaise*. Cover the sunburned parts with mayonnaise, store-bought or made from the recipe in the Glossary.
- *Oils*. Referred to as *sweet oil* in the 1800s, olive oil was applied to sunburned skin and covered with a light bandage. Polyunsaturated vegetable oils have greater skin-penetrating power and don't require bandaging.

  To make an oil and vinegar dressing: Cover the burned areas with vinegar-saturated cloths for 10 minutes, then remove the compresses and gently coat your skin with oil. For one-step application: Mix equal amounts of oil and vinegar in a shaker bottle.
- *Petroleum jelly*. Apply directly from the container or heat in the top of a double boiler until runny. If your skin is parched as well as sun-struck, place several layers of gauze over the petroleum jelly and cover with a heating pad (on its lowest setting) for 10 minutes to increase absorption.
- *Vegetable shortening*. In the 1940s, a standard remedy called for slathering a sunburn with white vegetable shortening and then turning round-and-round in the breeze from an electric fan.

- *Vinegar lotion* is a super-soother you can make ahead and store in the refrigerator.

  1 cup white vinegar

  1/3 cup *each* salt and yogurt

  2 tablespoons aloe vera gel

  400 IUs vitamin E from a snipped capsule

  Whisk or blenderize until creamy, transfer to a pump-dispenser bottle, then smooth over your uncomfortable skin every hour of so.

- *Vitamin E,* squeezed from punctured capsules or purchased in a bottle, is credited with relieving pain, transforming beet-red skin to bronzed-brown, and preventing the formation of blisters.

How to Heal the Blisters

When blisters erupt, the skin's protective barrier is damaged, and bacteria normally present on the outer skin quickly multiply in the plasma that leaks from the dilated blood vessels. The three cardinal rules for guarding against infection are

1. Wash blistered skin gently with mild soap and water.
2. Blot dry rather than rub with a towel.
3. Never attempt to deliberately open the blister by pricking or squeezing.

Covering the blisters with a protective coating of any of these substances speed healing:

- Aloe vera gel or petroleum jelly
- Avocado oil or wheat germ oil. To add healing benefits, blend 50,000 units of vitamin A and 1,000 IUs of vitamin E (obtained from punctured capsules) with 4 tablespoons of the oil.
- Honey or a half-and-half mixture of honey and wheat germ oil.
- Vitamin C (made into a liquid by dissolving 1 tablespoon of vitamin C crystals in 1/2 cup of water), or vitamin E from snipped capsules.

Dealing with the Leftovers:
Sun Spots and a Peeling Tan

Freckles and age spots often darken after exposure to the sun and become more obvious as a tan fades. Nutritionists and holistic doctors have found that the following supplements will help fade existing sun signs and prevent new ones from forming: B-complex vitamins with additional B-2, to lighten the spots;[74] vitamin C to build strong collagen that will prevent the pigment clumping that results in brown spots;[164] and vitamin E (100 IU with each meal) to forestall the instigating accumulations of melanin.[49]

Regardless of the care with which you cultivate a suntan, its demise is seldom a pretty sight. Filmy skin fragments detach themselves, departing blisters disclose pale patches, and you feel like a reptile shedding its skin. Fortunately, there are natural ways to speed a return to attractive normalcy.

How to wash off unsightly sun signs

Fifteen-minute tub-bath soaks followed by gentle rubbing with a washcloth or a loofah help to "wash off" no-longer-perfect tan by removing some of the darkly pigmented surface skin. Any one of these bath additives will hasten the process.

- *Milk or vinegar.* Add 2 cups of fresh milk (or 2/3 cup instant dry milk), or 1 cup of vinegar, to the bathwater to soften your skin, get rid of the dry flakies, and ease the separation of old, peeling skin from its fresh new replacement. Including a tablespoon of vegetable oil will leave your skin feeling satiny.
- *Lemon juice.* Add 3/4 cup strained lemon juice to your tub to lighten your skin and get rid of that flaky, last-rose-of-summer look.
- *Oatmeal.* Taking an oatmeal bath (as described for soothing a sunburn), then using the squishy bag as a scrubber leaves you with sleek, emollient-pampered skin.

Natural remedies for bleaching out uneven, fading tans

Centuries of insistence upon pale skin as an essential attribute of beauty have left us a legacy of natural remedies for bleaching out fading tans and brown sun signs.

Figure 10. During the 1890s, cosmetic preparations such as Mme. Ruppert's Face Bleach were popular

Borax is a skin-lightening favorite from the nineteenth century. Dissolve 2 teaspoons of borax in 1 cup of water. Add 1 cup of rubbing alcohol and 2 more cups of water, then sponge over your skin several times a day.

For a more potent remedy, mix 1/4 cup borax with 1/2 cup granulated sugar in a glass jar. Cover and let stand for 48 hours. Once each day, stir the mixture and rub a spoonful on your discolored skin.

"Glycerinated Lotion of Borax" was used as a daily wash to render the skin exquisitely soft and white. Mix 1 teaspoon powdered borax with 2 tablespoons glycerin and 3/4 cup rose water.

Botanicals have a well-established reputation for skin lightening.

Aloe vera gel. Smooth over sun-darkened freckles or brown spots at least twice a day.

Dry comfrey root tea. Mix to thick paste with water and apply to brown spots or splotches for 15 minutes each day. Rinsing off the paste with fresh lemon juice hastens the bleaching process.

Dandelion leaves. Liquefy a handful of the fresh leaves with three ice cubes in an electric blender. Strain before applying to discolored skin.

Dandelion flower and parsley lotion is reported to be even more effective. Bring 1 cup *each* dandelion blooms and chopped, fresh parsley to a boil in 4 cups of water. Cover and let steep until cool. Strain, refrigerate, and use the liquid as a wash two times a day.

Horseradish. Grate into buttermilk, vinegar, or water, then steep for several hours before straining and applying.

Watercress. Place a freshly washed bunch of watercress in 2 cups cold water. Bring to a boil, cover and simmer for 10 minutes. Strain and store in the refrigerator. Each morning and evening, sponge the chilled liquid over your fading tan, allow it to dry, then rinse with tepid water.

Fresh apricots, strawberries, and green grapes all have skin-bleaching properties. Use one of the apricot masques from Chapter 5, or simply mash the fruit and pat it on. For a more complex, but supposedly infallible fading-tan remover: Rinse a bunch of green grapes, sprinkle with a mixture of powdered alum and salt, wrap in parchment paper, and bake until tender. Squeeze out the juice and sponge it over your skin.

Cranberries contain acids that bleach and clear the skin. Once or twice each day, crush a handful of fresh or frozen cranberries. Rub the extracted juice over tanned areas, allow it to remain for several hours, then rinse off.

Lemon juice can be used in a variety of ways: Blended with an equal amount of glycerin, it can be sponged on to remove a tan. When mixed to a paste with salt or sugar and allowed to remain on the skin for half an hour once each day, lemon juice may lighten brown splotches caused by the sun.

Lemon juice and egg white. The 1870's instructions call for combining the juice of a lemon with the unbeaten white of an egg in an earthen bowl, placing it of the back of the stove for half an hour, and stirring constantly with an ivory spoon while taking care not to let the bowl get hot enough to crack. With modern appliances you can "cook" the mixture in a custard cup resting in a pan of boiling water over low heat on the rangetop, or microwave it on "defrost" until congealed. However prepared, it should be smoothed over the skin and allowed to remain for several hours.

Milk, in its many guises, is a time-tested skin lightener. Marie Antoinette bathed in buttermilk and spread sour cream over her face and shoulders to maintain her porcelain-white skin. In the 1890s, a tan-removing lotion was prepared by blending 1 cup milk, 1/4 cup lemon juice, 2 tablespoons *each* brandy and heavy cream, 1 teaspoon sugar, and a pinch of alum. The mixture was then brought to a boil, skimmed, and allowed to cool before being applied to the skin. (If this fails to do great things for your mottled tan, you might substitute nutmeg for the alum, omit the heating stage, and drink the concoction to improve your disposition!)

Yogurt, plain or blended half-and half with buttermilk, can be used as a night cream to ameliorate a fading tan.

Potato water is an old German cure for fading tans and summer freckles. Simply sponge on the water in which potatoes have been cooked.

Tomatoes. Mash ripe tomatoes and apply the pulp to your fading tan. Let dry before removing with water.

Section 2

Head to Toe Beauty

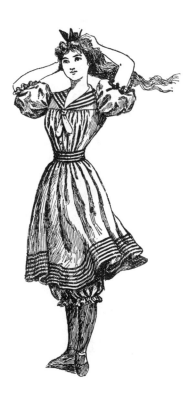

❧ 10 ❧

Handling Your Hands: Guidelines for Natural Nurturing

Exposed to public view more of than any other part of your anatomy except your face, hands should be attractive as well as functional; they can be disastrously revealing. Scarlett O'Hara's alluring "drapery dress" was a futile sacrifice; Rhett Butler discerned her subterfuge the moment he saw her work-worn hands. You needn't go to such extremes as sleeping with them tied above your head (an eighteenth-century Austrian method of maintaining small-veined, lily-white hands); natural nurturing can keep them at their best.

The Five-Minute Daily Workout
for Exercising and Massaging Your Hands

A brief daily workout increases blood circulation to your hands, strengthens their muscles and improves their flexibility.

1. Stand with your feet 12 inches apart; arms raised straight above your head. Keep your hands stiff while swinging your arms in windmill motions for a count of 20.

2. Sitting or standing, extend your arms parallel with your shoulders. Let your hands dangle loosely and shake them in a circular motion for 30 seconds.

3. With your elbows resting on a table, raise your hands and clench your fists. Open your hands, fan out the fingers and bend them backward as far as possible. Repeat 7 times. Slather on a generous coating of lotion. Grasp your left hand with your right, place your right thumb in the palm of the left hand, and the fingers of your right hand against the back of the left hand. Using deep but gentle circular motions, massage the palm, knuckles, and each finger. hange hands and repeat.

Tip: Gloves provide protection from dirt, detergents and water as well as cold temperatures. Unless you have coated your hands with lotion to give them a skin-softening treatment while washing dishes, waterproof gloves (even if fabric lined) should be removed every 15 minutes to allow your hands to breathe, and to prevent trapped perspiration from inducing chapping.

Natural Cleansers for Soothing Problem Hands

After removing any snug-fitting rings, moisten your hands, wash with a mild cleanser, rinse thoroughly, pat or blot dry. Neglecting these basics can result in "ring rash" or "ring rot," regardless of your jewelry's pedigree. A vacation shopper almost panicked when the skin under her new, half-inch-wide, sterling silver ring turned into a painful, leprous-looking, spongy white mass from an accumulation of public-restroom soap powder and lack of air. A film of vitamin E from a pierced capsule, plus air exposure, produced a quick cure, though prevention would have been more pleasant.

Sensitive or chapped hands

- Work a natural makeup-remover into your hands, tissue off, then rinse and blot dry. Or, smooth a facial masque over your hands and rinse it off as soon as it dries.

- Mix dry mustard (from the spice shelf), miller's bran, or oatmeal with water to make a paste. Rub it into your hands, then rinse off. If your hands are extremely sensitive, wash with oatmeal paste, then rub dry oatmeal over them to absorb the moisture.

- Soak your hands in a bowl of buttermilk, fresh milk, or rehydrated dry milk; or in a solution of mild shampoo and water; or in a mixture of sugar and water. Add a little uncooked oatmeal or miller's bran for additional soothing and softening.

Grubby, roughened or stained hands

The harsh abrasives in commercial heavy-duty cleansers often leave hands dry and irritated. Men and women will appreciate the gentle effectiveness of these natural cleansers.

- **Almond meal, cornmeal, or uncooked oatmeal**, mixed with water, heal as well as cleanse.

  Almond meal and honey, mixed half-and-half, massaged into hands and arms, steamed with hot towels for 5 minutes, and then covered with plastic wrap for 10 minutes before being rinsed off, provides cleansing plus soothing.

  Almond meal dairy cream is an eighteenth-century unisex cleanser-smoother you can store in the refrigerator for a month or so. Whip 1/4 cup almond meal with 2 cups milk. Bring to boiling over low heat and stir in a beaten egg yolk. Beat in 1 tablespoon almond oil and 1-1/2 teaspoons tincture of benzoin.

  Cornmeal is a great grease remover. Thelma was proud of Stan's ability to take care of maintaining their cars but objected to the aftermath of greasy doorknobs and "dirty" soap. Keeping a container of cornmeal in the garage solved their difficulties. Before he goes in to wash up, Stan wipes off as much of the grease or oil as possible, then removes the remainder by rubbing his hands with the cornmeal.

  Cornmeal and lemon juice or vinegar, blended to a paste, is an old stand-by for cleaning grimy hands that are roughened or chapped.
- **Ammonia water** (1 teaspoon ammonia per cup of water) is a highly recommended hand cleaner, but it must be followed by a moisturizer to prevent dryness.
- **Granulated sugar**, mixed to a gritty paste with water, is especially good for removing oil stains from hands.
- **Lemon juice or citrus peel** (scratched to allow the oils to seep out) removes surface discolorations.
- **Super Scrub**: If your hands are frequently grubby, keep a tightly covered jar of this mixture on hand. Combine 1/2 cup cornmeal with half of a grated 4-ounce bar of white castile soap, 2 tablespoons almond meal, (or 2 tablespoons dried lemon or orange

peel from the spice shelf), and 2 tablespoons almond or corn oil. Add more oil if needed to make a semisolid paste.

Natural Hand Lotions and Creams
That Moisturize and Protect

Hands have so few oil-secreting glands that the assistance of moisturizers is necessary to prevent dryness. To enhance the benefits of lotions and creams, smooth them on while your hands are slightly damp.

Glycerin, applied full strength, can draw moisture from the skin to dry it even further. Mixing the glycerin with rose water obviates the problem, as does blending 1 tablespoon tincture of benzoin with 1/4 cup glycerin, or stirring up a half-and-half combo of glycerin and fresh lemon juice.

Glycerin and hydrogen peroxide in equal proportions work miracles for abused hands.

Glycerin and rose water, the most widely known natural lotion, can be purchased from pharmacies or custom-made at home. The basic formula calls for 1 part glycerin shaken with 3 parts rose water. For a more potent mixture, combine 1/2 teaspoon borax with 1/2 cup rose water, then gradually stir into 1/2 cup glycerin. For a milder variation, blend 3/4 cup rose water, 1/4 cup glycerin, and 1/4 teaspoon *each* honey and apple cider vinegar.

Vinegar-flaxseed lotion is another time-tested remedy for uncomfortably dry hands: Soak 1/4 cup flaxseed in 2 cups water for 8 hours. Bring to a boil and simmer for 5 minutes. Strain. Add 1-1/2 cups apple cider vinegar and 1/3 cup glycerin to the liquid. Return to boiling and beat with a rotary beater to emulsify the mixture.

Grapefruit peel. Quarter half a grapefruit rind, rub the inner side of one piece over your hands; reserve the remainder in a plastic bag in the refrigerator.

Herbal lotions can be as simple as squeezing on the liquid from a camomile tea bag that has been soaked in 2 tablespoons boiling water for 2 minutes, or as complex as this *Herbal Unguent*: Combine equal amounts of angelica, basil, mint, pennyroyal, valerian, and stinging nettle in a small pan. Pour in white wine to cover the herbs; cook until they are tender and the wine almost boiled away. Mix in melted beeswax to make a thick salve.

Honey is a proven skin softener. For use as a hand lotion, reduce its stickiness by combining the honey with rose water and/or vegetable oil.

Lemon counteracts the alkalinity of soaps. Cook a chopped lemon in water to cover, whir the mixture in an electric blender, strain out any particles of peel, then smooth on the thick liquid.

Or, place a lemon slice in a small dish with 1/4 cup warm milk, cover and let stand for 3 hours. Strain off the liquid to use as a skin-smoother for hands and arms.

Or, blend 1 tablespoon *each* lemon juice, honey, and salad oil to smooth rough elbows as well as hands.

Milk, warmed and rubbed into the hands each night, dispenses with redness and soothes sore hands.

Oil lotion. Melt 1 tablespoon cocoa butter, stir in 1/4 cup almond oil, 2 tablespoons *each* olive oil and wheat germ oil, then blend in 1/4 teaspoon tincture of benzoin.

Petroleum jelly relieves roughened skin and is acceptable to males who resist fragrant cosmetic creams and lotions.

Vegetables. European peasants and American pioneers softened their hands with slices of raw cucumber or potato.

Vinegar. To restore the acid mantle and prevent parchmentlike dry skin, rub a few drops of apple cider vinegar into your damp hands after each washing.

Intensive Care Treatments:
Time-tested Secrets for Beautiful Hands

The age-old practice of applying a soothing unguent at night and wearing gloves to bed still works wonders for mistreated hands. White cotton gloves are as effective as the once-advised white kid. Wear them over a slathering of olive oil, petroleum jelly, any of the ointments described above, or one of these time-tested "secrets" for beautiful hands:

- **Banana butter.** Mash half a ripe banana with 2 teaspoons butter.

- **Egg-yolk salves.** Blend 1 teaspoon rice flour with a raw egg yolk. Stir in 2 teaspoons almond oil, 1 teaspoon rose water, and 1/4 teaspoon tincture of benzoin. Or, try this seventeenth-century chapped-hands remedy: Mix 1 tablespoon *each* honey, lanolin, and tincture of benzoin with 1 egg yolk and sufficient dry oatmeal to make a paste.

- **Lanolin**, originally called "wool fat," was prized as a cure for cracked and bleeding hands even before its prowess was praised in the writings of Ovid and Herodotus. Now stocked by pharmacies, pure lanolin can be used alone or mixed with almond or sesame oil in a ratio of 3 parts lanolin to 1 part oil. For an ointment, stir 2 tablespoons lanolin with 1 teaspoon petroleum jelly and 1/2 teaspoon tincture of benzoin. For a hand cream, mix equal amounts of lanolin and petroleum jelly. To smooth hands and elbows, and to overcome the ashy patches often besetting those with dark skin, blend 2 tablespoons each lanolin and vegetable oil with 1/2 teaspoon lemon or lime juice.

- **Mayonnaise,** either store bought or homemade (see Glossary for recipe), includes hand-soothing in its repertoire.
- **Potato cream.** Cook a small potato in its skin. Peel and mash with almond oil and glycerin to make a soft paste.

How to Have Fabulous Fingernails

Fingernail infatuation is not a recent fashion foible; long, beautifully groomed nails have been a status symbol in almost every period and culture. In 500 b.c., Queen Hetepheres was entombed with her manicure kit of seven golden knives and a metal "orange stick"; ancient Mandarins, who could barely lift a chopstick with their four-inch talons, guarded their nails with sheaths of gold, silver, or bamboo. Wearing today's artificial nails constantly can promote soft, peeling nails or trap moisture to cause moldy fungal infections. Helping Mother Nature grow your own is safer and less expensive.

Tips on nourishing your nails

Nails appear bonelike but are composed primarily of protein (one-fifth of their structure is fluid, another fifth, fat) and derive their nourishment from blood vessels in the dermis. The *matrix* (growth portion) extends beneath the exposed nail bed, produces nails at the rate of about 3/16 inch per month, requires up to six months to grow a new nail, is speedier in summer than in winter, slows with age, and is influenced by nutrition and general health as well as external care. Studies of nail texture as a means of detecting marginal malnutrition have led to the discovery that internal nail-nourishment requires a daily minimum of 60 grams of protein[32]—much more than an occasional infusion of gelatin (which is helpful if its missing amino acids have been supplied with milk or meat broth) plus a well-balanced diet and supplements when needed.

- *B-complex combination.* Taking a B-complex stress tab plus garlic perles and a zinc supplement each day is said to duplicate the fantastic fingernail improvement achieved by a month of treatment at a European health spa.[19]

- *Brewer's yeast,* 1 or 2 tablespoons per day, encourages nail growth—especially when accompanied by calcium supplements.

- *Calcium,* 1,200 milligrams per day (the amount in a quart of milk), is a healthy-nails essential.

- *Iodine* is another requisite for nail health and strength. Salmon, tuna, iodized salt or a kelp salt-substitute are natural sources.

How to care for your nails

Six to eight daily glasses of water (or their equivalent) are vital for nail health. (As explained in *Health,* January 1988, brittle, flaky nails can result if their moisture level drops below 18 percent.) Too much external water, however, leads to a variety of nail problems. To avoid oversubmersion, rest your hands on the sides of the tub while luxuriating in your beauty bath, and wear rubber gloves for dishwashing or household cleaning. When your nails are water-logged, applying hand lotion or petroleum jelly will help seal in the moisture to prevent damage. If you are about to embark on a gloveless, grubby project, plan ahead by digging your nails into a bar of soap. After your chore is concluded, remove the soap and grime with a nailbrush. Other external encouragements include:

Buffing with a chamois buffer to improve circulation, promote growth, and add sheen. Buff gently from cuticle to tip; buffing too vigorously, or with back-and-forth motions, can build up heat and harm your nails. Massage a bit of petroleum jelly or wheat germ oil into your nails before buffing to help strengthen them. For a conditioning treatment that imparts an amber tint, try the "hennicure" once favored by Egyptian royalty. Make a paste from 1 teaspoon dry henna and water. Rub a thin coating into your nails and let it dry before buffing. If you would rather not have the coloring, use neutral henna.

Exercising them by playing the piano, embroidering, doing needlepoint, typing, even tapping your fingers to stimulate growth. Just don't abuse your nails by assuming they are screw-tighteners or tile-grout cleaner-outers.

Filing your dry nails from the outside toward the center with an emery board or diamond file. (A steel file or vigorous seesawing may trigger nail splitting.) Use nail clippers or scissors only after your nails have been softened by soaking.

Nourishing them from the outside. Soak your unpolished nails for 10 minutes in a bowl of warmed almond oil (or other natural oil) to which you have added the contents of a vitamin E capsule. Wipe off the excess but do not wash your hands before going to bed.

Or, mix 1 tablespoon wheat germ oil with 1 tablespoon honey, 1 egg yolk, and 1/8 teaspoon sea salt. Massage into your nails each night and wash off each morning. Store the mixture in the refrigerator between treatments.

Four ways to care for your cuticles

Cuticles help prevent bacteria from attacking the nail base. Protect them by rubbing in a dab of petroleum jelly before swimming or putting your hands in soapy water, cut them only if a hangnail develops, and keep them attractive by:

- Pushing them back with a towel, cotton-tipped swab, or an orange stick each time you clean your hands.

- Massaging them every night with cocoa butter, petroleum jelly, or vitamin E from a snipped capsule.

- Removing roughness by soaking them in warm oil for 5 minutes, then rubbing them with almond meal or cornmeal.

- Trimming off the loose skin of a hangnail, then coating the area with fresh lemon juice, petroleum jelly, or vitamin E from a pierced capsule.

Natural Remedies for Nine Common Fingernail Problems

Nails, although hard, are extremely permeable to water or other fluids. According to the *Harvard Medical School Health Letter* of May 1984, water moves through a fingernail 100 times faster than it penetrates the outer layer of skin. Lengthy immersion disrupts nail structure by causing them to expand with moisture, then shrink as they dry; and may instigate ridging, splitting or breaking. When detergents or household chemicals are added to the water, nails are further weakened and damaged; studies in Great Britain confirm actual loss of fingernails due to detergents.32 If nail problems have developed, there are natural remedies and treatments.

1. **Brittle, splitting nails** can result from prolonged exposure to water; insufficient dietary protein, calcium, sulfur, zinc, or vitamins A, B, and C;

chronic illness or stress; oral contraceptives; nail polish or polish remover (adding a few drops of olive oil or castor oil to the remover, and washing your hands immediately after its use, helps counteract the drying effect).

Brewers's yeast and choline. Taking 2 tablespoons of brewer's yeast in a glass of juice or milk plus 1,000 milligrams of choline each day improves nail strength.

Iron. A deficiency can cause dry, brittle fingernails. Increasing your intake of iron-rich foods (see Vitamin and Mineral Chart) and taking vitamin C to boost assimilation of the iron may resolve the problem.

Oil treatments are a standard remedy. Soak your polish-free nails in warm wheat germ oil (or other natural oil) for 5 to 10 minutes each day, then massage from the tips toward the cuticle. Dr. Robert W. Downs, writing in *Bestways* (January 1986), suggests gently breaking the nails' surface tension with an emery board to allow better penetration of the oil.

Soda. Once each day, dissolve 1 tablespoon baking soda in 1 cup of water for a 10-minute fingertip soak. Follow with an application of air-excluding oil or lotion.

Vinegar. Nightly soaks in a half-and-half mixture of apple cider vinegar and warm water are a folk remedy for splitting nails.

White iodine, applied over the tops and under the nail tips twice a day, does more than discourage nail nibbling—it helps restore fingernail flexibility and strength.

2. **Discolorations and stains** can be caused by illness, prolonged stress, or by contact with chemical contaminants such as carbon paper, hair dye, nail hardeners or polish, or cigarette smoke. If the nail plate is deeply stained, it will remain so until the new nail grows out. To remove surface stains: rub them with a cut lemon, or wiggle your fingertips in a lemon half, then rinse and dry.

3. **Misshapen nails.** Artificial fingernails have been found responsible for upward curving nails.[161] Spoon-shaped or flattened nails can result from long-term protein or iron deficiencies, and may be remedied with improved diet.

4. **Opaque nails** with a wavy pattern may indicate a lack of protein, a shortage of vitamin A or B, or a mineral imbalance. Improving your diet and supplementing it with a multivitamin plus extra B-6 and 15 milligrams of zinc each day may correct the problem. Totally white nails may indicate a liver disorder; check with your physician.

5. **Pale nails** may be a sign of low zinc and B-6, or can be caused by anemia. See your doctor if the condition persists after you've upgraded your diet.

6. **Pitted fingernails** may indicate a deficiency of calcium, protein, or sulphur (available from eggs, garlic, and meats).

7. **Ridges, grooves, and furrows** can result from careless cuticle trimming or from wearing artificial nails, but usually are caused by illness or nutritional deficiencies.

Horizontal ridges (Beau's lines) often occur following severe stress or illness. Eating an adequate diet with ample protein, and taking supplements of vitamin C plus 15 milligrams of zinc each day, speeds their growing out and disappearing.

Vertical furrows can indicate a deficiency of vitamin A, calcium, or iron. Sometimes they simply begin to develop after the age of 40 because of reduced cell reproduction and are no cause for concern as long as your annual checkup reveals no anemia or lack of vitamins and minerals.

8. **Soft, weak nails.** Excessive contact with water or the chemicals in nail cosmetics are the most common cause; stress and faulty diet come next. Munching on sunflower seeds, increasing your intake of vitamin A (see Vitamin and Mineral Chart), taking 5,000 milligrams of dolomite (a calcium-magnesium supplement reported to restore thin, fragile nails to normalcy in three weeks[175]) and a 15-milligram zinc tablet daily, or swallowing 1 teaspoon of apple cider vinegar three times a day are other successful remedies. Although fingernail formation depends on internal nourishment, beveling your nails so there are no blunt edges discourages peeling. There are other strengthening treatments:

Apple cider vinegar or white iodine. Smooth over polish-free nails with a cotton-tipped swab.

Henna. Prepare the neutral shade for a conditioning nail-dunk. Soak your fingertips for 5 minutes, then rinse, dry, and apply hand lotion or a vegetable oil.

Horsetail. Steep 1 tablespoon of the dried herb in a cup of boiling water until comfortably warm. Use as a nail-soak for 10 minutes each day. To increase the benefits, herbalists advise swallowing a tablespoonful of the hot brew each morning and evening.

Oat straw. Drinking a cup of oat straw tea every day is the folk healer's prescription for improving fingernails.

Oil soaks restore fingernail strength by providing or reinforcing the fat content of the nails. Any vegetable or nut oil may be warmed for the purpose; the addition of vitamins A and D, or E (from snipped capsules) makes the soaks more effective. Whenever possible, indulge in a 10-minute oil soak at bedtime, tissue off the excess, then refrain from washing your hands until the next morning.

9. **White spots** are the most intriguing nail problem because they are attributed to everything from telling fibs or acquiring a new sweetheart to being deficient in zinc and vitamin B-6. Folklore utilizes them as a fortune-telling medium with this rhyme for counting the white spots:

A gift, a ghost, a friend , a foe,

A letter to come, a journey to go

Injuries, particularly from cuticle removing, have been known to cause white spots; so have estrogen medications, extreme cold, fasting, fungus infections, and menstrual cycles.

Dr. Pfeiffer[127] and other holistic practitioners correlate all of these occurrences (except for the recent boyfriends, falsehoods, future prognostications, and blows to the nail matrix) to low levels of zinc—so a daily 15-milligram zinc supplement may be worth a try if you have white spots in your fingernails. Or, you can experiment with Dr. Jarvis' folk-medicine remedy of stirring 1 teaspoon *each* apple cider vinegar and honey into a glass of water to accompany each meal.[84]

ૐ 11 ૐ

Putting Your Best Feet Forward: Special Remedies & Exercises for Your Sole Protection

Feet are less vulnerable to signs of aging than other body parts, and don't acquire bulges if you gain a few pounds, but they do grow weary. And they are entitled to. During a lifetime they travel a distance equaling three times the circumference of the globe, withstand 1,000 tons of pressure each day as the average worker or homemaker walks a daily ten miles, and support 200 tons of stress when a 125-pound person runs one mile.[128] Until our Cro-Magnon ancestors forsook walking on all fours, body weight was more evenly distributed; the millenia required for evolutionary adjustments, plus almost constant use, account for the tiredness radiating form our overworked feet.

How to Feed Your Feet

To perform their amazing feats, the 26 bones in each foot (one-fourth of all our bones are in our feet) must be nourished internally by calcium (at least 1,200 milligrams per day plus accompanying magnesium, phosphorus and vitamin D), and the muscular structure of our pedal extremities must be maintained with adequate protein, vitamin C, and potassium. (See Vitamin and Mineral Chart for food sources.)

124

Protecting Your Feet: Practical Tips for Selecting Shoes

Foot traffic in prehistoric villages tamped walkways into unyielding surfaces that were uncomfortable for bare feet accustomed to grassy meadows, so shoes were designed solely for sole protection. By 2,000 B.C., Egyptians were cushioning their feet with sandals woven from reeds. Ancient Romans wore leather half-boots or wooden shoes: Northern Europeans enclosed the toes with fur for warmth. Practicality, however, soon gave way to the dictates of style. In the fifteenth century, courtiers supported the 18-inch turned-up toes of their slippers with chains attached to their waists, and aristocratic ladies elevated themselves on 30-inch-high platform-soled shoes called chopinnes. (So many miscarriages resulted from pregnant women toppling off these "stilts" that a law prohibiting such dangerous footgear was passed in Venice in 1430.)

Fortunately, current fashion lacks these extremes. *Footwear News* reports that sales of walking shoes rose 72 percent during 1988, and comfort has become a major concern. Witness the numbers of business-women wearing tennies to commute to work!

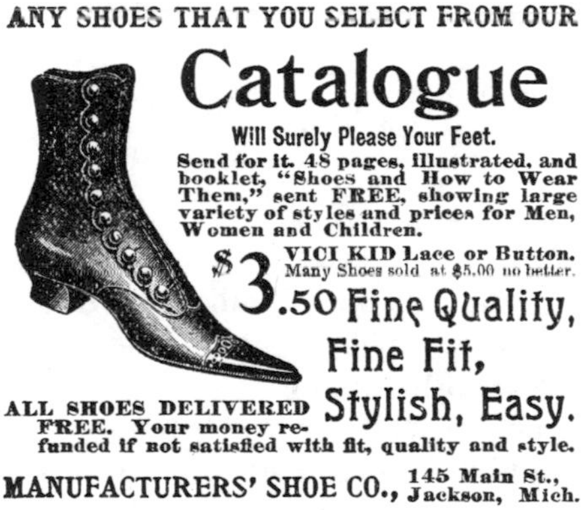

Figure 12. American gentle-women of the 1890s compressed their feet into stylishly pointed shoes, then stuffed the toes with crumpled paper to prevent rubbing holes in their stockings.

Statistics appearing in *Hippocrates* (November/December 1988) reveal that 45 percent of women wear uncomfortable shoes, and, according to the American Podiatry Association, improperly fitting shoes are the most common cause of the over 30 million podiatric visits made annually.[6] Here are some sensible guidelines to follow:

- Don't go shoe shopping in the morning. That perfect fit at 10 a.m. may put frown lines on your face by 5 p.m. because feet expand by as much as half a size during the day.

- While standing with your weight on one foot, check the space in the "toe box" by wriggling your toes and pressing down on the shoe. There should be a quarter to a half inch of space beyond your longest toe.

- Boot heels should slip a little, shoe heels should neither slip nor sag. Calf-hugging boots should not be tight enough to restrict circulation after a few hours of wear.

- When trying on shoes, wear hosiery suited to the footwear (sports socks require shoe space) and be sure the clerk understands your intended use of athletic shoes. The steel-plated soles of biking shoes can do you in if you wear them for jogging; aerobic-dance shoes will not provide the support you need for hiking.

- Double check the fit of your new shoes when you get home by pulling a pair of old socks over them (to avoid soiling the soles) and walking around for an hour. If you notice any discomfort, exchange the shoes. Otherwise your feet may break down before the shoes are broken in.

Exercises That Benefit Your Feet and Ankles

Physical activities that benefit the rest of the body usually involve the feet and ankles, yet provide them little relief.

Hi-heeled compensation

Mother Nature never intended for us to walk on tiptoe with our feet thrust forward by the force of high heels—the higher the heel, the more unnatural the position. Besides instigating possible postural problems, wearing high heels can cause the hamstring muscles behind your calves to atrophy from not being stretched as far as if your heels were touching the ground.

Ellie was so conscious of her diminutive height that she wore 4-inch heels to work and high-heeled bedroom slippers at home. Enrolling in a fitness program brought her down to earth. She was ready to cancel during the first session; performing the required movements on tiptoe was impossible, and lowering her heels to the floor was too painful. Ellie's coach suggested she gradually stretch her calf muscles with these exercises:

1. Stand 3 feet away from a wall, lean in and place your hands against the wall, stretching them as high as possible. Holding your arms

straight and your heels flat on the floor, push into the wall for a
count of 15. Repeat 10 times.

2. While standing with your feet 12 inches apart, rock back and forth
    by lifting first your toes and then your heels off the floor. Intensify
    the effect by raising your arms high over your head as you rise on
    your toes, lowering your arms as you rock back on your heels.

3. Fold a towel lengthwise to a 4-inch width. Sit on the floor with legs
    straight out in front, knees stiff. Loop the towel under your toes
    and pull back to stretch each calf 6 times.

After a few weeks, Ellie was able to walk comfortably in athletic
shoes and rejoin her class. To forestall future difficulties, she stretches her
hamstrings each evening, and wears low-heeled shoes or slippers during
her hours alone.

Relaxation and strengthening techniques

Regardless of shoe-heel-height, if foot muscles are not in shape,
inflammation and ankle sprain can result. Walking helps improve circulation and prevent nighttime cramping. To help prevent other foot and
leg problems, elevate your feet whenever possible, vary heel height from
day to day, and exercise your feet regularly.

- Sit in a chair, hold your feet above the floor with heels down,
  then make arcs from left to right like windshield-wiper blades.

- Spread a towel on the floor. Stand on it and scrunch it up with
  your toes.

- Use your toes to pick up pencils or marbles, or to turn the pages
  of a phone book, one at a time.

- Climb the walls. Lie flat on the floor with the soles of your feet
  propped against a wall. "Walk" slowly up and down the wall
  by grasping with widespread toes.

- Stand with feet turned out to approximate 10 minutes to 2 on a
  clock face. Walk forward for 10 steps, backward for 10 steps.
  Repeat with the toes turned inward like clock hands set at 20
  minutes before 4.

- Walk barefoot on a yielding surface—beach sand or thick car-
  peting—as often as possible. Barefoot trodding of city pave-
  ments or public swimming-pool decking is not recommended.
  Besides being uncomfortable, these surfaces are rife with contaminants that can lead to foot infections.

Arch supporters

- Roll a rolling pin, a 12-ounce beverage can, or a tennis ball under your bare feet for several minutes each day.

- Stand on tiptoe, throw your weight to the outside of your feet, and come down slowly. Then walk on the balls of your feet for 30 seconds. Repeat the routine three times.

- Each morning, before putting on your shoes, stand with feet flat on the floor, then rise on your toes with a springing motion. Repeat 10 times.

- When you get home at night, take off your shoes and tiptoe around the house for 3 to 5 minutes. If truly "foot weary," reduce the walking time to 2 minutes, then sit on the edge of the bathtub and run warm water over your feet for 2 minutes; follow with 1 minute of cold water.

Flat-foot foilers

- To prevent or relieve the pain of flat feet: Squat with your weight on your toes, then slowly rock backward until your weight is on your heels. Repeat several times. If necessary, steady yourself by holding onto a stable object.

- Stand with toes pointing inward in a pigeon-toed position. Go up and down from toe to heel 15 to 20 times.

How to Revitalize Your Feet with a Massage

Foot massage stimulates blood circulation, which is important not only for your feet, but also for facial attractiveness and the well-being of the rest of your body. You can use a hand lotion (see Chapter 10) for massaging your feet, or mix up a jar of this *Lubricating Massage Oil* to share with your tired-footed mate: Melt 1 tablespoon lanolin in the top of a double boiler. Stir in 3/4 cup peanut oil and 1/4 cup olive oil. Add 1/4 cup rose water and emulsify with a rotary beater.

Malcolm's first day as a postman was too much for his feet. He hobbled to the parking lot, removed his shoes, and was sitting with his feet propped up on the dashboard when a co-worker paused to initiate him into the rites of foot massage. "Rub some life into those dead dogs," advised the kindly veteran.

1. Grasp the sole of one foot with both hands, thumbs against the heel, and gradually massage toward the toes.
2. Place your thumbs on top of the foot next to the ankle and massage forward to the toes.
3. Play "this little piggy" by gently rotating and pulling each individual toe.
4. Repeat with the other foot.

The relief was so miraculous that Malcolm repeated the massage at lunchtime for a few days. Now, a veteran himself, he merely revives his feet each evening.

For a traditional Chinese massage to revitalize your feet:

1. Rotate your ankles while massaging each toe.
2. Massage the soles of your feet with your fists.
3. Rub the tops of your feet from ankles to toes in circular motions with the flat of your hand.

For a pressure massage to relieve swollen, tired feet:

1. One at a time, hold each toe with your thumb and index finger and apply firm pressure on three spots: the cuticle, the toe joint, and the base of the toe.
2. Massage the spaces between the toes, then move up the instep toward the ankle.
3. Place both thumbs under one heel and massage forward to the ball of the foot, then back to the Achilles' tendon. Repeat with the other foot.

For a quick massage to stimulate your feet: Place a layer of dried peas or beans in a pair of low-heeled oxfords and walk a few steps—very few, any more would be painful.

How to Soak Out the Wearies:
Five Natural Solutions for Adding to Your Footbath

When you don't have time for a beauty bath, invigorate your feet by rubbing them with a lemon wedge or by sitting on the edge of the bathtub and running cold water over them for a few minutes. Better yet, soak them for 10 minutes in a foot tub or dishpan that will hold enough of one of the following solutions to reach your ankles. Rinse if necessary, dry thoroughly, then lightly massage with peanut oil or a moisturizing lotion.

- **Coffee grounds.** Refrigerate your coffee grounds so they won't sour, then utilize their remaining tannic acid to revive your feet. Boil 1 cup of the grounds in 2 cups water for 5 minutes. Strain into your footbath and add cool water.

- **Epsom salt.** Place 3/4 cup epsom salt in your footbath. Swish with hot water to dissolve, add lukewarm water for a comfortable soak, then rinse with cold water.

- **Herbs.** Brew double-strength tea with camomile, comfrey (dried leaves or roots), horsetail, lavender, mint, or sage, then strain into the footbath.

- **Salt.** Using 2 foot basins and alternating soaks of hot salt water (1/2 cup table salt in an ankle-high basin) for 3 minutes with 1-minute cold-water soaks for 2 repetitions (conclude with the cold) gives exhausted feet a new vigor.

   Salt and soda, 1/4 cup *each* table salt and baking soda, dissolved in warm water, soothe and smooth.

- **Vinegar and lemon.** Swish 1-1/2 cups cider vinegar and 1/2 cup fresh lemon juice with tepid water.

How to Take the Heat Out
of Burning Feet

Burning sensations on the soles of the feet may be due to a deficiency of B-complex vitamins. Taking extra B-5, B-6, and B-12 along with a daily multivitamin often resolves the problem within a few weeks.

For instant relief, try a circulation-stimulating mustard footbath prepared with dry mustard, or cook up an old-fashioned *Bran Bath:* Stir 3 cups miller's bran into 4 cups cold water. Bring to boiling, cover and let stand for 10 minutes. Strain into your footbath. Add cool water and 1/4 cup baking soda. Soak your feet for 15 minutes. You can reserve and reuse the bran-soda solution each night for a week.

Good Old-fashioned Cures for Those Aching Feet

1. **Bandage them with onions.** Roast whole onions until soft; discard the outer layers; mash or puree the onions and apply to the feet on a cloth bandage.

2. **Bury them in sand.** Fill a deep pan with sand; add boiling water to make it moist and warm; bury your feet for 30 minutes and add more hot water if the sand cools too quickly.

3. **Soak them in oak bark tea.** Steep double-strength tea from red or white oak bark. Soak your feet for 15 minutes each night and morning.

4. **Wrap them in cabbage.** Remove the hard central ribs from a dozen large cabbage leaves. Soften the leaves in the top of a double boiler or in a covered container in the oven. Fold the warm leaves around your feet and cover with towels or plastic bags for 15 minutes.

Natural Remedies for Correcting
Seven Common Foot Problems

Athlete's foot

Medically referred to as *tinea pedis*, the term "athlete's foot" was coined in the 1930s to glamorize a foot-powder promotion. The problem never was limited to athletic males (a university survey shows that 15 percent of the female students have athlete's foot[132]) and it is not as contagious as formerly believed. It can, however, be transmitted via shed fragments of affected skin, and can spread to moist skin folds in the pubic area or armpits, to the nails or the scalp. The infection may be caused by any of several species of fungi or by various types of bacteria that thrive on moist warmth, and are triggered or worsened by emotional stress, physical illness, or air-excluding footwear which can increase the cup-per-day of moisture normally excreted by the feet. Daily cleansing with thorough drying (particularly between the toes), and wearing "breathable" shoes, are both preventives and treatment. If the painful "itchies" have established a foothold, try a natural remedy:

- Supplement your daily diet with a multivitamin, a B-complex tablet, 1,000 milligrams vitamin C, and 400 IU vitamin E; and take 2 acidophilus capsules or eat a serving of yogurt with each meal.

- Wear silk hosiery or acrylic socks to draw perspiration away from your feet. The once-advised white cotton socks absorb moisture and hold it close to the skin.

- Remove athletic shoes immediately after perspiration-producing activities; wear leather sandals whenever possible.

- Bathe your feet with a mild alcohol or vinegar rinse twice a day to restore the pH balance disturbed by the infection.

- Soak your feet once daily in a solution of 1 tablespoon salt per quart of water; or in a footbath of golden seal tea, thyme tea, or a combination of camomile and thyme tea.

- Powder your feet with cornstarch to help absorb moisture and reduce friction; or dust them with powdered golden seal as a curative.

- Apply aloe vera gel every morning and evening, or smooth on yogurt at bedtime and wash it off in the morning. Or, try a B-vitamin ointment made by mixing pulverized B-2, B-3, and B-5 tablets into a paste with brewer's yeast and sesame oil.

- Coat the affected areas twice daily with this variation of the "Wonder Cream" used by Russian soldiers: Blend 2 tablespoons lanolin and 1 tablespoon cod liver oil with 1-1/2 teaspoons *each* garlic powder and honey.

- Expose your feet to sunlight for a total of 1 hour each day in 20-to 30-minute sessions.

Blisters

Massaging your feet with glycerin before wearing new shoes may help prevent blisters. Experienced hikers recommend wearing ankle-high silk or nylon hose under thick orlon, cotton, or wool socks. If a blister does form: avoid the source of injury, protect the blister from further harm with a cushioned bandage, then allow it to heal naturally without pricking. Applying garlic oil (squeezed from a garlic-perle supplement) under the bandage is a modern folk remedy for relieving the pain of a blister and speeding its healing.

Bunions and bunionettes

Bunions (projections from the base of the big toe) and bunionettes (on the little toe) may be hereditary, but customarily result from a combination of loosening ligaments and constricting footwear. If the bunion does not push out too far, it may be corrected by eating a nutritious diet to strengthen the supportive muscles, padding with protectors, rubbing with a little pulverized saltpeter dissolved in olive oil, or with this 1890s treatment: Add 1 tablespoon ammonia per quart of hot water for a footbath. After a 10-minute soak, grasp your foot with one hand. With the other hand, pull your big toe away from your foot and gently rotate it under the water. Reheat the water and soak for another 10 minutes. Dry your feet, then paint the bunion with iodine.

Calluses and corns

Dietary deficiencies may be responsible for a proclivity toward calluses (thickened areas of skin formed by the body to protect the flesh over bony prominences) and corns (conical overgrowths with hard, central cores resulting from abrasion or pressure). Including more vitamin A and potassium in your diet (see Vitamin and Mineral Chart) may help circumvent them. Eliminating friction and pressure by wearing well-fitting shoes should prevent their regrowth. Padding around calluses or corns offers temporary relief from the pain they engender; removal usually can be accomplished by one of these natural methods.

1. Soak your feet in soapy water or a solution of hot water and baking soda or dry mustard or salt, or in any of the footbaths suggested for other foot problems. After the soak, gently rub the callus or protruding corn with a pumice stone (smoothing on a coating of glycerin before using the pumice makes it more effective). Blot dry and coat with lotion, petroleum jelly, white vegetable shortening, or a mixture of 2 tablespoons vegetable oil and 1 teaspoon cider vinegar.

2. Massage aloe vera gel, castor oil, or vitamin E from pierced capsules into the calluses or corns twice each day; or, rub them with a paste of baking soda and water.

3. Walk on sand. Joanne's job as a sales rep required a lot of pavement pounding in fashionably high-heeled, thin-soled shoes, and the calluses her feet developed in self-protection were becoming painful. When she realized that walking barefoot on the sandy shore while vacationing had restored her feet to callusless comfort, Joanne put a beach in her bathtub for year-round "foot vacations" to prevent a discomforting recurrence. She keeps a shallow container of sand in the bathroom, places it in the tub after each bath or shower, and "marches in place" for a few minutes. Then she rinses and dries her feet and massages them with lotion.

4. Try a folk remedy for removing corns: Make a paste with breadcrumbs and cider vinegar, or with baking soda and petroleum jelly; apply to the corn each night until it can be lifted out.

Or, each night for a week, cover the corn with the cut half of a raw cranberry, a slice of raw garlic, the pulp side of a small piece of lemon, a bit of raw onion, or a paste of onion cooked in vinegar.

Or, bind cotton over the corn and saturate it three times daily with turpentine.

Or, every other day, soak the corn-containing foot in a solution of hot water and dry mustard, rub the corn with vinegar, then dry and apply a touch of white iodine.

5. Soft corns between the toes may be mollified and prepared for removal by sponging with rubbing alcohol or castor oil, then wrapping the adjoining toes with wisps of wool yarn; or by scraping a piece of common white chalk, placing a pinch of the powder on the corn and binding it in place with a strip of soft cloth.

Dry, rough, or flaky feet

Before going to bed, soak your feet for 15 minutes in warm, sudsy water (use your favorite soap or shampoo) to which you have added baking soda or oatmeal. Rinse and dry; massage with castor oil, peanut oil, or petroleum jelly; then sleep in a pair of old socks.

Linda's feet were neither callused not corned, but her heels felt rough and had a dirty gray cast. The night before the beach party, she decided something must be done. After her beauty-bath-soak, she scrubbed her heels with a nail brush, thoroughly dried them, rubbed in vitamin E from pierced capsules, and covered them with bed socks. The gray roughness disappeared, and, to her delight, stays away as long as she gives her heels a weekly vitamin E treat.

If only the bottoms of your feet are afflicted; sprinkle a layer of table salt in a shallow pan, dampen it slightly and slide your feet back and forth. Rinse, dry, and massage with lotion or oil.

If your legs as well as your feet are flaky, transform them into glossy gams with one of these treatments: Sit on the edge of the bathtub and run warm water over your legs and feet. Blot off the excess water, coat the skin with honey or molasses, then read or meditate for 30 minutes. After rinsing and drying, rub in a half-and-half mixture of lanolin and olive oil.

Or, exfoliate your legs and feet with one of the facial scrubs from Chapter 2. Rinse, dry, apply a moisturizing oil or lotion, then cover with plastic wrap for half an hour.

Foot odor

Try supplementing your diet with 30 milligrams of zinc every day, placing a spoonful of dry oatmeal or miller's bran in your socks, or experimenting with one of these naturally deodorizing, moisture-absorbing foot powders.

- Baking soda and cornstarch, mixed half-and-half.
- One-fourth cup *each* cornstarch and fuller's earth, mixed with 2 tablespoons zinc oxide.
- One-half cup cornstarch mixed with 1/4 cup zinc oxide and 1 tablespoon powdered orrisroot. Sprinkle 1 teaspoon of the mixture in each shoe.

Ingrown toenails

To avoid toenail edges growing into adjoining soft tissue, cut the nails straight across and smooth them with an emery board or diamond file. Do *not* cut a "V" in the center of the nail. Besides being ineffectual and painful, this self-inflicted torture can instigate additional problems.

If an ingrown nail is caught before it becomes infected, home treatment is usually effective. After each shower, tub bath, or footbath, gently insert a wisp of cotton under the offending nail corner. To increase the benefit, soak your foot in a solution of hot water and epsom salt, then saturate the cotton with castor oil or vitamin E from a snipped capsule before tucking it under the nail edge. A folk-remedy alternative is a salve made from laundry soap, thick cream, and granulated sugar.

❧ 12 ❧

Smiling Pretty:
How to Care for
Your Mouth & Teeth

What with food consumption and oral communication, mouths are in motion even more than feet. As sources of beauty and expression as well as functional necessities, they are justifiably entitled to a fair share of any beauty and health regimen.

Protect and Soothe

Although lips are constantly being stretched, puckered, and exposed to moisture and extreme temperatures, they contain no oil glands. To prevent (or to heal) dry, chapped lips, follow the beauty experts' advice to "never let your lips go naked" by coating them with honey, lemon juice mixed half-and-half with glycerin, oil, petroleum jelly, or one of these lip protectors and soothers.

Natural lip gloss and pomade

In the top of a double boiler (or in a heat-proof dish in a pan of boiling water), stir 1/4 cup petroleum jelly into 2 tablespoons melted beeswax or paraffin. Or, beat 5 tablespoons vegetable or nut oil into 1 tablespoon melted beeswax or paraffin. Or, blend 1 tablespoon honey with 1-1/2 tablespoons melted beeswax or paraffin, then beat in 2 tablespoons vegetable oil. Remove from the heat and stir until cooled. Store the pomade in tiny pillboxes or jars. If it becomes too hard, reheat over hot water and stir in a few drops of vegetable oil.

You can add color to your lip gloss while it is still warm by stirring in food coloring or a teaspoon of alkanet root (which produces a lovely burgundy shade but should be strained through gauze after mixing).

Do-it-yourself remedies for lip problems

Chronically dry, sore lips may be due to a cosmetic allergy, a deficiency of dietary fatty acids, or to an internal yeast infection. If going without lipstick (or switching to a hypo-allergenic brand), including two tablespoons of vegetable oil with your daily meals, and experimenting with Mother Nature's lip smoothers fail to bring relief, check with your physician.

- Coat your lips with honey or petroleum jelly after every washing and before bed each night. Or, blend 4 teaspoons glycerin with 1 teaspoon tincture of benzoin and smooth over your lips several times a day.

- Sponge triple-strength white oat bark tea over your lips 3 times a day.

Cracks at the corners of the mouth (*cheilosis*) may result from an allergy to commercial mouthwash or toothpaste, from overindulgence in alcohol or spicy foods, or from B-vitamin or fatty-acid deficiencies. A shotgun-approach of avoiding questionable foods and products, taking a high potency B-complex tablet with each meal, and drizzling a tablespoon of vegetable oil on each salad should resolve the problem.

Cold sores and fever blisters are caused by *herpes simplex virus 1*, which lurks in a dormant state and can be activated by stress, menstrual difficulties, sunburn, or any illness with a fever. The sores and blisters may spread to the inside of the mouth as canker sores. Toothbrushes are a haven for the virus. If you have a cold sore, switch to a new toothbrush when the blister breaks and again after it has healed. Rather than wait for these unappealing abominations to run their course, try a natural remedy:

- *Acidophilus*, ingested in the form of capsules or tablets taken with milk 4 times a day, or as a generous serving of acidophilus yogurt with each meal, usually relieves local soreness within 24 to 48 hours.[23]

- *Aloe vera gel* from a freshly cut plant contains antibacterial, anti-fungi substances that are lacking in the commercially stabilized gel. Application of the gel at the onset often forestalls cold sores.

- *B-complex vitamins,* taken in high-potency tablets twice daily, may abort an incipient cold sore. Early cures and shortened durations have been achieved by adding 100 milligrams of niacinamide; by taking 500 milligrams of B-5 every two hours; or by combining the B-5 treatment with twice-daily doses of 50 milligrams B-6, 350 micrograms B-12, and 500 milligrams vitamin C with bioflavonoids.

- *Herbal treatments*: Sponge triple-strength red clover tea over the cold sore several times daily. Or three times a day, sip a cup of hot sage tea into which you have stirred a teaspoon of powdered ginger.

- *Ice.* Holding a chip of ice against an erupting sore may halt its development.

- *Lysine* (an amino acid available without prescription) is credited with rapid cures when 1,000 milligrams are taken daily. Lysine is even more miraculous when combined with the acidophilus therapy described above.

- *Salt water and brandy.* At the first sign of a fever blister, dissolve all the salt possible in 1/4 cup of boiling water. Apply to the sore with a cotton ball every hour, then sponge with brandy.

- *Vitamin C,* accompanied by a calcium supplement and taken in 150 to 1,000 milligram doses each hour, helps clear cold sores.

  When Gordon's cold sore erupted the weekend before he was to present the ad campaign he'd worked on for months, he had to do more than speed its recovery—he had to make it disappear. Hoping to augment the effectiveness of the vitamin-C therapy, he coated the blister with vitamin E from a pierced capsule before patting on the powdered C. Every hour, after taking his tablets of calcium and vitamin C, Gordon reapplied the topical treatment. The strategy worked. His lip was still tender, but no lip-puffing sore marred his successful presentation.

- *Zinc,* ingested daily as a 30 to 150 milligram tablet, or pulverized and applied directly to cold sore, is another blister-banisher.

How to Nourish Your Teeth

Inert as they seem, teeth are alive. Composed principally of calcium, phosphate, and protein, they constantly renew themselves with nourishment from their roots in the bloodstream and the minerals washed over them by saliva. They, and their support, must be strong and healthy to withstand the up to 200 pounds of pressure exerted by the jaw muscles when we chew. A well-balanced diet, including adequate protein and calcium, is essential; a daily multivitamin-mineral supplement provides insurance against possible deficiencies.

- Lack of vitamin A can lead to tooth decay.
- Vitamin C deficiency can cause degeneration of tooth enamel, weakened supporting tissues, and bleeding gums.

Extremely hot or cold foods or drinks can cause dental enamel to suffer "thermal fatigue," which can lead to the formation of fissures in the teeth, and, not only what we eat but when we eat it, affects dental health:

- Chewable vitamin C, sweets, or sweetened beverages should be indulged in at mealtimes (not between meals) so the acids left in your mouth will be neutralized.
- Starches and fats can be as harmful as sweets. An enzyme in saliva transforms starch into sugar; fat makes food stick to the teeth. Raisins and peanut butter are among the worst offenders; most damaging of all is the folk practice of taking a spoonful of blackstrap molasses as a before-bed sleep-inducing nostrum.
- Chocolate, nuts, and certain cheeses (Cheddar, Monterey Jack, Swiss)help neutralize the decay-causing acids.
- Eating a quarter of a raw apple after a meal removes 30 percent more food debris from the teeth than an immediate brushing.[99]
- Taking 1 teaspoon of apple cider vinegar stirred into a glass of water at each meal is a folk remedy for reducing plaque and strengthening gums.
- Chewing sugar-free gum or ginger root, or rolling your tongue around your mouth to simulate tooth brushing, activates the salivary glands to protect the teeth and relieve a dry mouth.
- Drinking generous amounts of tea (which contains flouride) provides as much protection from tooth decay as flouridated

water. In *The Food Pharmacy* (Bantam 1988), Jean Carper recommends using tea as an anti-cavity mouthwash.

Sturdy foods such as crispy salads, nuts, seeds, and whole-grain toast not only provide excellent nourishment; they also stimulate blood circulation to the teeth and gums, and lessen the risk of periodontal disease (which affects 90 percent of adults, accounts for all but 2 percent of tooth loss, and gives rise to bad breath and bleeding gums). Munching hard candy, ice chips, or popcorn kernels can crack your teeth. Chewing unchewable substances can wear them down; witness ancient skulls with teeth abraded to half their original length by the grit included with flour ground on stone metates.

How to Message Your Gums and Protect Against Gum Disease

The friction of direct massage helps preserve a tight collar af gingival tissue around the teeth to protect against gum disease.

- Lightly brush the gums with a soft-bristled toothbrush, or use the flexible rubber tip on the handle of your brush.
- Make a paste of baking soda and 3 percent hydrogen peroxide. Rub this into the gums with a fingertip, then rinse your mouth with a saline solution of 1/4 teaspoon table salt in 1/4 cup water.
- Massage your gums with table salt, then rinse with water.
- Several times each day, practice the Oriental pressure-massage of pressing the corners and the center top and bottom of the lips with a firm, rotating motion.

How to Cleanse Your Teeth

An inmate of England's infamous Newgate Prison devised the first toothbrush by inserting tufts of hair into a piece of bone drilled with tiny holes. Prior to this ingenious invention, teeth were cleansed by chewing on twigs, rubbing with cloth, or by having the debris poked out of their crevices with toothpicks of porcupine quills, ivory or gold, or with the pointed ends of eating knives. The origin of our round-tipped dinner knives is attributed to Cardinal Richelieu's edict prohibiting the sharp tips that so often drew blood when seventeenth-century diners picked their teeth.

Directions for which direction to brush with what type of bristles at which angle have undergone radical changes since "up and down with stiff bristles" was eulogized. The most recent advice from the American Dental Association is to use a brush with soft, rounded bristles, hold it at a 45-degree angle to the gum line and brush in a slow circular motion, covering about three teeth per circle. To reach the inside of the front teeth, insert the brush vertically and gently push it up and down; then brush the chewing surfaces with short back-and-forth strokes.

For controlling plaque and removing debris between the teeth, correct flossing is as vital as brushing. Curve the dental floss around each tooth and scrape up and down several times, then employ a gently sawing motion between the gums and the neck of each tooth.

When to Clean Your Teeth

Concluding each meal with a few bites of fibrous food (apple, orange, raw carrot, or celery) and a "swish and swallow" mouth-rinsing of plain water is considered as effective as brushing every time you eat. In fact, according to a report in *Health* (October 1987), one thorough cleansing per day may be all that is necessary because mouth bacteria require 24 hours for recolonization. Periodontists, however, still advise brushing every 12 hours for plaque control. The most important time to clean the mouth is the last thing at night to prevent sugar molecules or food particles from wreaking their havoc during sleeping hours.

How to care for artificial teeth

The first false teeth were clumsy contraptions carved from ivory and held together with metal springs (George Washington's famous "falsies" were made from walrus tusks, not wood). Later experiments with celluloid proved unsuccessful because of the inflammability, as exemplified by public catastrophes in which smokers' dentures caught on fire. Whether with "partials" or full dentures, the mouths of more than half the population over 45 are now enhanced with artificial teeth, which, regardless of formulation, require daily cleansing to prevent tartar build-up and unpleasant breath. It is especially important to remove partial dentures for cleaning to avoid a collection of food fragments in the recesses around retention clips.

If the sensitive tissue around or beneath artificial teeth becomes tender, rub your gums with aloe vera gel or vitamin A (squeezed from a pierced capsule) and supplement your diet with 30 to 100 milligrams of zinc daily until the soreness disappears.

How to deal with discolored teeth

Depigmentation, white spots, or a mottled appearance may be the result of childhood exposure to overly flouridated water, illnesses with high fevers, prescriptive doses of tetracyline, or deficiencies of vitamins A, B, or E. Dr. Ronald T. Maitland, 1988 spokesperson for the American Dental Association, warns that abrasive pastes and polishes set up a vicious pattern of roughening and wearing away tooth enamel to make teeth more prone to staining.

Recently acquired surface discolorations from coffee, tea, acidic foods or beverages, or from smoking, that remain after normal brushing and flossing may be removed by brushing with baking soda; rubbing with a fresh strawberry; or by scrubbing with lemon peel, then thoroughly rinsing with water.

Natural Dentifrices:
Four Natural Cleansers for Fighting Germs and Plaque

Many dentists believe dentifrices serve only to add piquancy to the otherwise boring task of tooth cleaning. This is borne out by studies of over 50 different brands of toothpaste—none proved more effective at preventing dental caries than proper flossing and brushing with plain water[115]—and, although several flouride-containing dentifrices have acceptance as cavity fighters, *Parade Magazine* (February 7, 1988) reports that no toothpaste or gel has the American Dental Association seal for plaque removal.

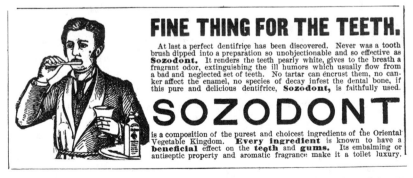

FINE THING FOR THE TEETH.

At last a perfect dentifrice has been discovered. Never was a tooth brush dipped into a preparation so unobjectionable and so effective as **Sozodont.** It renders the teeth pearly white, gives to the breath a fragrant odor, extinguishing the ill humors which usually flow from a bad and neglected set of teeth. No tartar can encrust them, no canker affect the enamel, no species of decay infest the dental bone, if this pure and delicious dentifrice, **Sozodont,** is faithfully used.

SOZODONT

is a composition of the purest and choicest ingredients of the Oriental Vegetable Kingdom. **Every ingredient** is known to have a **beneficial** effect on the **teeth** and **gums.** Its embalming or antiseptic property and aromatic fragrance make it a toilet luxury.

Figure 13. The recorded formula for this liquid dentifrice, marketed in 1893, shows little of benefit, or of Oriental origin: 10 ounces water, 4 ounces honey, 2 ounces alcohol, 1/2 ounce potassium carbonate, with sufficient oil of rose and oil of wintergreen to flavor.

In 1860, borax, dissolved in water, was suggested for destroying the parasitic mites believed to exist in remnants of food fermenting between the teeth. During the 1880s, beauty conscious ladies were advised to brush their teeth with white soap instead of harsh dentifrices, and were assured that the slightly unpleasant taste would soon pass unnoticed. In lieu of laundry products, there are other natural cleansers:

- *Apple juice or lemon juice.* Brush, then rinse with water.
- *Baking soda* has none of the silicates contained in abrasive dentifrices, and, long before modern dentists began recommending it for stain removal, soda was combined with other natural substances for cleaning teeth, killing germs, and preventing plaque.

  Mix equal amounts of soda and sea salt; mix 1/2 cup soda, 1 tablespoon sea salt, and 1 teaspoon ground cinnamon; mix 1/2 cup soda, 1/4 cup dried lemon or orange peel (pulverized in an electric blender or coffee grinder), and 4 teaspoons table salt; or, make a paste with soda and a mashed strawberry or 3-percent hydrogen peroxide.

Herbal tooth powders

- *Black walnut* powder, brushed on the teeth, is credited with restoring tooth enamel.[144]
- *Mint leaves, Peruvian bark, and rosemary leaves,* lightly roasted and ground to a powder with charcoal, cleanse and polish teeth.

25 Herbs You Can Use to Make Your Own Natural Mouth Rinses

The Federal Drug Administration has found most ingredients in commercial mouthwashes useless; many unsafe.[128] For easily prepared, natural "mouth rinses," steep one to three ounces of any of the following herbs (singly or in combination) to make double-strength tea. For germ-fighting benefits, soak the herbs in 2/3 cup ethyl alcohol (or 80-proof vodka) for one week; strain and dilute with 1-1/3 cups distilled water.

Agrimony: astringent, good for receding or bleeding gums, promotes healing after tooth extraction

Angelica root: relieves pain, promotes healing

Anise seeds: aromatic flavoring, relieves pain

Camomile: reduces gum inflammation and pain, aids healing

Cardamom: freshens breath, used as flavoring

Catnip: relieves mouth soreness

Cinnamon: freshens breath

Cloves: freshens breath, kills germs, reduces pain

Comfrey: astringent, good for bleeding gums, relieves pain

Eucalyptus: antiseptic

Fenugreek: freshens breath, relieves mouth inflammation

Golden seal: astringent, antiseptic (has an antibiotic action similar to Tetracycline and Streptomycin)

Horsetail: freshens breath, strengthens tooth enamel

Lemon balm: freshens breath, relieves mouth soreness

Myrrh: antiseptic, astringent, aids bleeding gums and mouth inflammation

Peppermint and *Spearmint*: antiseptic breath fresheners, promote healing

Plantain: helps bleeding gums, reduces pain and mouth inflammation

Rosemary: freshens breath

Sage: strong astringent, reduces saliva production, folk remedy for bleeding gums

Sandalwood: astringent, disinfectant

Shave grass: reduces bleeding, improves healing and prevents scarring after dental surgery

Thyme: scientifically proven antiseptic which gives a famous mouthwash its characteristically unpleasant flavor

White oak bark: astringent, relieves canker sores, strengthens gums, helps set loose teeth

Winter savory: scientifically confirmed antiseptic

Witch hazel bark: relieves soreness and bleeding gums

Three easy antiseptic mouthwash recipes

1. *Food flavorings (extracts)*. Shake 1 to 2 tablespoons extract with a mixture of 1/2 cup *each* ethyl alcohol (or 80-proof vodka) and distilled water. Use almond to soothe pain; lemon for bleeding gums; peppermint, spearmint, or vanilla for flavor; wintergreen for killing germs, reducing pain, and strengthening gums.

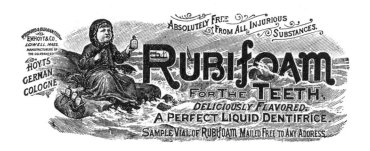

2. *Mint flavored.* Soak 1/2 teaspoon *each* crushed cloves, myrrh, thyme, and spearmint in 3/4 cup ethyl alcohol for 1 week, shaking the bottle daily. Strain, add 10 drops oil of peppermint and 1-1/2 cups distilled water.

Or, combine 1 cup *each* ethyl alcohol and distilled water with 1 teaspoon *each* peppermint and wintergreen oil.

3. *Nonalcoholic.* Boil hyssop leaves in vinegar to cover, strain, and use as a rinse to relieve a sore mouth.

Or, steep 1/4 teaspoon *each* of anise, mint , and rosemary in 3/4 cups boiling water for 10 minutes. Strain and use as a rinse for bleeding gums or an irritated mouth.

Or, combine 2 tablespoon *each* dried eucalyptus leaves, lemon balm, peppermint, plantain, sage, and thyme. Boil 4 teaspoons of the mixture in 1 cup water for 10 minutes. Let stand, covered, for another 10 minutes. Strain and bottle for an all-purpose mouthwash.

How to Banish Bad Breath

The most obvious case of unpleasant mouth odor is strongly flavored food such as garlic or onion. Eating the fresh parsley or cilantro often served as a garnish with halitosis-generating meals; chewing cloves, cardamom or dill seeds, or chlorophyll-thymol tablets from health food stores are convenient away-from-home breath purifiers.

Less obvious is the fact that fragments of food lurking between the teeth may cause even the blandest of meals to create offensive mouth odors. The 98.6-degree temperature in the mouth instigates the decomposition of bits of meat, eggs, and similar foods within a few hours. When you neglect to sequester a few bites of fibrous veggies to munch on for teeth cleansing after dessert—and immediate brushing is not feasible—hie yourself to the powder room and clear the crevices with a toothpick.

Brushing your tongue each time you brush your teeth reduces mouth odor 60 percent more effectively than just brushing and flossing your teeth;[80] rinsing with mouthwash adds the finishing touch. If that combination plus these natural remedies does not resolve the problem, visit your dentist and physician to be sure decaying teeth, kidney dysfunction, or digestive problems are not responsible.

- Eat acidophilus yogurt every day, or take acidophilus supplements with each meal.
- Rinse your mouth two or three times a day with equal parts of horseradish and honey diluted with water. Or, swish with triple strength tea made from equal amounts of golden seal, myrrh, and rosemary.
- Drink a cup of fenugreek, peppermint, or rosemary tea each morning and evening. Add 1/4 teaspoon anise, cinnamon, cloves, or mace to each cupful to increase the efficacy of the tea.
- Drink 2 cups a day of this Breath Freshening Tea:

  2 tablespoons *each* anise, camomile, lemon balm, and peppermint

  1 tablespoon *each* angelica root, cloves, echinacea, and dried parsley

  Soak 1 teaspoon of the dry mixture in 1 cup cold water for an hour, bring to a boil, cover and steep for 5 minutes, then strain.

❧ 13 ❧

Watching Out for Your Eyes: How to Relieve Eyestrain & Other Common Ailments

When it comes to creating a first and lasting impression of beauty, the eyes have it. Romantic poets refer to them as windows of the soul; pragmatic physicians believe they mirror the state of physical health. Regardless of how others view our eyes, their well-being is essential if we are to see out of them. Sunglasses help prevent damage from ultraviolet rays; goggles guard them while we gaze at underwater wonders or work with equipment that might produce flying fragments; wearing collars with room for two fingers between fabric and neck allows an ample supply of nutrient-bearing blood to reach them. (A study at Cornell University revealed that 67 percent of the white-collared males tested were suffering from eye impairment due to restricted circulation from too-tight collars.)

How to Nourish Your Eyes

What we ingest has a profound effect on our eyes. Thirty-five hundred years before vitamins were "discovered," Egyptian physicians successfully treated night blindness with ox liver, and in 500 B.C., Hippocrates was prescribing raw liver (2 ounces = 30,000 IUs of vitamin A)

147

for his patients with dimming sight. Vitamin A has been acknowledged as the "eye vitamin" since World War II fighter pilots dined on carrots (26,000 IUs of vitamin A per cup) to restore their night vision. Although excess vitamin A stored in the liver can be harmful, there is little danger of toxicity from the vitamin-A precursor, beta carotene, in foods or supplements because the body converts it to vitamin A only as needed. Good vision also depends on a well-balanced diet and a constant supply of vitamins B, C, D, E, and the minerals calcium and zinc (see Vitamin and Mineral Chart for food sources). Daily amounts recommended by nutritionally oriented ophthalmologists:

A: 10,000 to 30,000 IU

B complex: 25 milligrams of each of the major B vitamins

C: 1,000 to 4,000 milligrams in divided doses

D: 400 to 1,000 IU

E: 100 to 400 IU

Calcium: 1,200 to 2,000 milligrams

Zinc: 15 to 50 milligrams

Studies conducted by the U.S. Department of Health, Education, and Welfare have established that smoking reduces visual acuity, color perception, and night vision, by decreasing the amount of oxygen delivered to the eyes by the blood vessels. Taking additional vitamin C (25 milligrams per cigarette smoked) and extra B-2 (30 to 50 milligrams plus a daily B-complex supplement) helps nullify the adverse effects of nicotine and carbon monoxide. Other recent findings link eye disorders to specific dietary overindulgences: alcohol blurs vision by interfering with the optic nerve; animal fats, refined carbohydrates and sugars, and excess salt adversely affect vision by altering the viscosity of fluid within the eye and changing the focal length of the eye's refraction. An excess of refined sugar also depletes calcium and chromium from the elastic cells in the eyes, causing the eyes to stretch out of shape and lose their normal focusing ability.[70, 94]

Drinking a glass of water containing 2 teaspoons *each* apple cider vinegar and raw honey at each meal is a folk remedy credited with maintaining good eyesight.[84] Eating raw fruit and vegetables benefits the eyes by providing enzymes necessary for vitamin and mineral assimilation, and a daily glass of any of the following mixtures is reported to improve vision in two weeks.[118, 179]

3/4 cup carrot juice + 1/4 cup spinach juice.

2/3 cup carrot juice + 1/4 cup celery juice + 1 tablespoon spinach juice.

2/3 cup carrot juice + 1/4 cup green lettuce juice + 1 tablespoon cod liver oil.

1/2 cup carrot juice + 1/2 cup celery juice.

Techniques for Reducing Eye Fatigue and Increasing Muscle Strength

Quick-start morning massage

Including a brief eye massage in your morning beauty routine improves circulation to distribute nourishment to the eyes, helps eliminate any puffiness, and gives you a youthfully wide-eyed start on the day.

1. Dab oil or cream on the under-eye skin. Put the first two fingers of your left hand one-half inch from the outside corner of your left eye; pull to the left to slightly tighten the skin. With your right index finger, start under the inside corner of your left eye and massage around it with gentle, circular movements. Change hands and repeat with the other eye.
2. Place your index fingers on the lower eye sockets, one-half inch from the outside corners of the eyes. Press and massage for 10 seconds.
3. Press the index finger of each hand under the center of each eyebrow. Close your eyes and rest the second finger of each hand on the eyelid. Try to open your eyes against this gentle pressure. Relax and repeat 5 times.
4. Open your eyes wide. With your fingertips, push up on your forehead just above each eyebrow for 5 seconds. Relax and repeat 5 times.

Six simple eye calisthenics

Like all muscles, those controlling eyeball movement grow stronger with exercise, and tire if held in a fixed position too long. Interspersing eye calisthenics with periods of visual concentration lessens eye fatigue and increases the strength of these six pairs of orbital muscles.

- Hold your index finger about 10 inches in front of your eyes. Look at the tip of your finger, then look into the distance. Repeat 10 times.

- Look steadily at an object on the wall while slowly rolling your head in a circle. Close your eyelids and slowly roll your eyes in clockwise, then counterclockwise, circles. Repeat 5 times.

- Without moving your head, look up, down, left, and right, as far as possible. Dart quick glances at the corners of the room. Close your eyes for 5 seconds, then repeat.

- Blink both eyes as fast as you can 15 times. (Blinking exercises two other sets of muscles: sphincter muscles that contract when you close your eyelids, another pair that raises the lids.) Wink one eye at a time while keeping the other eye open, 10 times for each eye. Tensing the entire face on the same side as the wink helps prevent bagging or dark circles under the eyes.

- Open your eyes as wide as you can. Slowly roll them in a circle to the left, then to the right. Close your eyes for 5 seconds between each of 5 repetitions.

- For a complete regimen, try this variation of Yoga therapy for improving eyesight and relieving eyestrain:

  1. Sit upright. Slowly nod your head 3 times toward your chest, your left shoulder, your back, and your right shoulder.

  2. Slowly roll your head clockwise, then counterclockwise.

  3. Inhale with your eyes tightly closed; exhale, open your eyes and blink rapidly 10 times.

  4. Without moving your head, move your eyes in a slow circle to the left, then to the right. Look diagonally toward the corners of the room, then up and down.

  5. Vigorously rub your hands together. Close your eyes, cover them with your palms, and take 5 slow, deep breaths.

"Palming": The Best Way to Rest Your Eyes

"Palming," first introduced by Dr. William H. Bates,[74] is still considered the best way to relax tired eyes.

1. Sit comfortably in an armchair or at a table with your elbows supported. Close your eyes and cup your palms over them without touching the eyelids.

2. Relax and take slow, deep breaths until the restful gray you "see" with your closed eyes turns into velvety blackness.

3. Open your eyes and blink rapidly a few times.

Getting the Red Out: Five Natural Solutions for Bathing Your Eyes

Many strange substances have been use to cleanse and refresh eyes, get the red out, and relieve the feeling of grit behind the eyelids. Inserting drops of castor oil, milk bottled with a white poppy, or a wash made with dried hen's dung were once popular. For added sparkle, Spanish senoritas squeezed the oil from orange peel into their eyes and colonial Americans "flirted in" soapsuds; both mistreatments seemed effective because the irritation causes the eyes to form tears to wash away the discomfort.

Human tears are Mother Nature's prescription for bathing the eyes. To simulate tears, use filtered sea water (purchased in bottles at health food stores), or a saline solution made from 1/4 teaspoon salt dissolved in 1/2 cup water. Folk practitioners suggest dissolving 2 tablespoons of clean rock salt in 1 quart of rain water (or bottled water), then immersing the face and blinking the eyes several times to wash the eyes and clear redness; or using one of these natural eye washes and drops:

1. **Baking soda**: 1/2 teaspoon dissolved in 1/2 cup water.
2. **Herbal teas**, made from 1 level teaspoon of dried herb steeped in 1 cup boiling water and well strained.

   Borage helps clear redness and relieves stinging from cigarette smoke or wintry winds.

   Camomile relieves watery or inflamed eyes, and speeds healing of eye infections.

   Elderflower clears redness.

   Eyebright cleanses the eyes and improves sight.

   Fennel, prepared from powdered seeds and strained through a paper coffee filter, refreshes weary eyes, reduces inflammation or watering, and is suggested as a twice-daily eyebath for glaucoma or other ocular diseases.

   Golden seal, lemon grass, red raspberry, or *sassafras teas* may be used as either drops or washes to relieve eyestrain and refresh the eyes.

   Pekoe tea, 1 teaspoon of the brew diluted with 1/4 cup water, may be used for either drops or baths to relieve eye irritation resulting from hay fever.

3. **Honey.** Stir 1/2 teaspoon into 1/2 cup lukewarm water.

4. **Milk.** A few drops of milk will relieve eye irritation caused by grains of salt or pepper. Equal parts of milk and water or strained sassafras tea may be used for refreshing eye drops or washes. For sore eyes, try this eighteenth-century potable eye bath: Boil 4 ounces camomile tea in 2 cups milk until reduced to 1 cup. Dissolve 2 tablespoons brown sugar in the hot liquid, stir in 1/2 cup rum, strain and bottle.

5. **Rose petal water.** Boil unsprayed, fresh rose petals in water to cover. Strain into a sterilized bottle for use as eye drops or baths to strengthen the eyes and relieve irritation caused by hay fever.

Nine Soothing Compresses and Poultices for Refreshing Tired, Irritated Eyes

When using eye compresses or packs, reclining, (preferably on a slantboard) for 10 to 15 minutes enhances their benefit. Wet tea-bag compresses are one of the most effective ways to refresh tired, itchy, puffy, or watery eyes. Make-ahead pads of cotton saturated with witch hazel and stored in a jar in the refrigerator are even more convenient.

1. *Alum water.* Saturate eye pads in a solution of 1/8 teaspoon alum and 1 cup water.

2. *Beets,* cooked, chilled, grated, and sandwiched between pieces of gauze, help relieve eyestrain. Direct application of raw cucumber slices is equally effective.

3. *Bread.* Toast and cool a slice of stale bread. Cut in half, soak in ice water, then wrap in cloth for eye compresses.

4. *Herbal poultices*: Borage, camomile, elderflower, eyebright, fennel, hyssop (by itself or mixed half-and-half with St. John's wort), rose hip, sassafras, slippery elm, verbena, or witch hazel bark in moistened tea bags (or compresses of wet tea leaves wrapped in cloth.)

5. *Golden seal tea* brings relief to tired eyes. Steep 1/4 teaspoon of the dried herb in 1/2 cup boiling water. Cool, strain, then use to saturate eye pads.

6. *Milk,* warmed to room temperature and used to saturate eye pads, puts the sparkle back in weary eyes.

7. *Orange juice,* freshly squeezed and strained, then used to moisten gauze pads, is an eye refresher.

8. *Papaya-mint* or *plain papaya tea bags* soaked in hot water, then chilled, not only refresh tired eyes but also reduce under-eye bags.
9. *Potato,* hand-grated or processor-pureed, raw potato wrapped in gauze is a time-tested remedy for tired eyes and sandy eyelids.

Natural Remedies for Six Common Eye Problems

Black eyes

Apply an ice pack or a cold compress (soft-pack frozen veggies are fine, but raw beef steak is no longer advised) for 15 minutes once each hour for 4 or 5 hours. Or, boil hyssop leaves, slippery elm bark, or soapwort roots until tender, wrap in gauze and secure over the eye at bedtime. Do not remove until morning.

Bloodshot eyes

Capillary weakness resulting from deficiencies of vitamin C and bioflavonoids may be responsible for redness that does not clear with natural eyedrops and baths. If the problem continues after dietary supplementation of 5,000 milligrams vitamin C plus 1,000 milligram bioflavonoids daily, consult your physician—allergies or conjunctivitis might be the cause.

Dark circles or bags beneath the eyes

These beauty detractors may not be due to either debauchery or illness. Under-eye tissue is so fragile that pockets can develop as repositories for fat or fluid, and is so transparent that the veins may show through as dark shadows.

- Compresses of moist camomile, pekoe, or rose hip tea (or warmed castor oil or olive oil) help remedy the problem if left in place for 15 minutes to several hours daily.
- Placing half a fresh fig or a poultice of grated raw cucumber under each eye for 15 minutes each day has been effective in some cases.
- Nighttime "fluid pooling" may be responsible for morning puffiness; try sleeping with two extra pillows tucked under your head. Or, freeze babies' teething rings, wrap in soft cloth, and place over your eyes for a few minutes.

Droopy eyelids

- For immediate, temporary relief, chill 2 teaspoons in ice water and place them over your closed eyelids.

- If weakened muscles are the cause, increase your dietary protein and add supplements of vitamin C, bioflavonoids, and vitamin E. Then strengthen the miniature muscles with exercise. Several times daily, cup your palms over your eyes and stretch the eyelids upward and outward for 10 seconds. Or, squeeze your eyes tightly shut; slowly relax the squeeze and lift your eyebrows, stretching the lids upward as far as possible without opening your eyes. Relax and repeat 5 times.

- Lids swollen from fluid accumulation may respond to 50 milligrams per-day supplements of vitamin B-6 plus compresses of moist camomile or pekoe tea bags.

Dry eyes

Inadequate nutrition or lack of humidity in desert-dry air or overheated rooms may instigate itching and burning not caused by allergy or eyestrain. An improved diet with daily supplements of 300 milligrams of Omega-3, plus frequently misted house plants or a humidifier, help moisturize eyes as well as skin. More often, dry eyes result from failure to blink as often as we should to keep our eyes lubricated. To remedy the problem, take a 10-second "break" of rapid blinking while changing focus from near to far during close work, deliberately blink at the end of each line of reading material, and use natural eye drops or washes every day.

Eyelid lumps and inflammations

Sties (tender bumps and little abscesses that suddenly bulge out between the roots of the eyelashes) and *chalazions* (slower-growing cysts that form on the edge of an eyelid when a gland inside the lid becomes plugged) usually can be cleared with natural remedies.

- Saturate a lint-free cloth (or gauze eye pads) with hot water and hold against the sty for 10 to 15 minutes at a time, 3 or 4 times daily.

- A moistened pekoe tea bag, or a compress of warm castor oil or dampened baking soda wrapped in cloth and left in place overnight, often drives away burgeoning sties by morning.

- A persistent sty can be treated with a poultice of grated raw potato, which may bring it to a head so it will burst and dissipate.

Blepharitis, eyelid inflammation with crusting and scaling at the base of the lashes, is related to abnormally increased dandruff and often contains infectious bacteria. If natural eye drops and dandruff treatments (see Chapter 14) do not resolve the problem, professional care should be sought.

How to Cultivate Long, Luxurious Lashes

Each lash has an individual life cycle consisting of a six-month growth period followed by a resting period during which it separates from the root so a new lash can form in the follicle. A few eyelashes are dislodged daily by washing or rubbing the eyes, and the unnoticeable process continues. The massive lash-and-brow fallout sometimes engendered by severe malnutrition or lengthy illness is usually followed by regrowth after good health is regained.

Cutting off your lashes in the hope of having them grow in longer and thicker doesn't work, but there are natural means of encouragement that have proven successful:

Castor oil or olive oil. A nightly brushing with either of these oils is an old-fashioned, slow-but-sure treatment practically guaranteed to produce long, silky eyelashes.

"Huile de Ricin," an exotic sounding French formula for luxurious lashes, can be duplicated by adding a sliver of lemon peel to the small bottle of oil used for daily brushing.

Liquid protein, sold as a dietary aid, strengthens and lengthens eyelashes when brushed on nightly.

Petroleum jelly, applied each night and morning, helps correct brittle, breaking eyelashes and makes them appear longer.

Vitamin D. Each evening, snip a capsule of vitamin D and pat the contents over your lids and lashes. Fantastic results have been reported after less than three months of this treatment.[32]

How to Beautify Your Brows

Eyebrows should compliment your face and accentuate your eyes, not attract attention to themselves. To encourage growth and thickening, rub lanolin or any of the eyelash-stimulators into the brows each evening before bed. If your eyes are close set, removing a few extra hairs from the inner edge of the brows can give you a more wide-eyed appearance; otherwise, brows should begin directly above the inner eye corners. Besides plucking the stragglers under and between your eyebrows, you may want to adjust their shape to conform to your facial structure.

Arched if your face is round.

Rounded if your face is heart shaped.

Slightly arched if your face is square or rectangular.

Straight if you have a long slender or oval face.

To eliminate tweezing discomfort when removing superfluous hairs, and to leave the vacated skin smooth and attractive:

1. Wipe your brows with an alcohol-or astringent-saturated cotton ball to remove any traces of oil.
2. Brush your brows the "wrong way" with an eyebrow brush or child's toothbrush to clear out any leftover makeup or flaky skin, then stroke them back into place.
3. For ouchless plucking: press an ice cube over the area for a few seconds, blot with a tissue, then tweeze one hair at a time in the direction of hair growth.
4. Finish by again wiping the area with alcohol or astringent, then apply a moisturizer or a coating of honey. The honey not only softens the skin, it acts as a natural bactericide.

Overly thick, bushy eyebrows (masculine or feminine) can be trimmed with manicure scissors or thinned with tweezers. To train your eyebrows and keep them in line: start by brushing them straight up on your forehead, then coax them into the proper shape with the side of the eyebrow brush. Smoothing on a dab of petroleum jelly or hair-styling gel while brushing will help keep them in their place.

❧ 14 ❧

Hair Care:
Tips on Controlling,
Conditioning, & Coloring

Crowning glory and face framer, hair shelters our heads from heat, cold, and injury. It has held an aura of fascination since fairy-tale Rapunzel lowered hers as a ladder for her lover, Lady Godiva made her famous ride, and wasp-waisted nineteenth-century ladies piled so much of it under their hats that they had to perambulate with out-thrust bosoms and bustled buttocks.

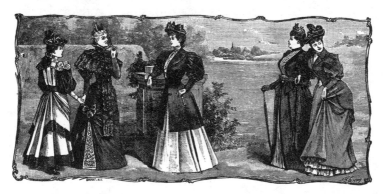

Hair grows approximately one-half inch per month until it reaches a length of 10 to 12 inches, then growth slows to half speed. After a three-year *anagen* (growing) phase, cell production ceases for three months (the *telogen* or resting phase) while replacements are formed. The inner core of the hair receives nourishment from blood vessels in the scalp. The outer layer (the *cuticle*) is composed of overlapping scales that, when hair is well cared for, lie flat to seal in natural oils and reflect light from our shining tresses. When internal supplies are inadequate, or when external abuse roughens the outer layer, dull, lifeless-appearing hair results.

How to Nourish Your Hair

Healthy hair depends on a nutritionally sound diet. Protein deficiencies can halt the growth phase, causing hair to shed prematurely. Excessive amounts of sugar, refined carbohydrates, or alcohol, can deplete the B-for-beautiful-hair vitamins. Smoking robs the body of vitamin C and constricts the supply-carrying blood vessels. In addition to iodized salt or kelp salt-substitutes to furnish iodine, suggested hair enhancing daily supplements are 1 multivitamin-mineral, 25,000 IU vitamin A in the form of beta carotene, 1 B-complex stress tab, 1,000 milligrams vitamin C, and 15 to 30 milligrams of zinc.

Do-It-Yourself Scalp Massages That Stimulate Blood Flow

A tight scalp restricts the flow of nutrients and prematurely moves hair into the preparing-to-fall-out stage. If your hair is oily, massage gently. If it is dry, massage more vigorously to stimulate the oil glands. For a quick daily massage, use your fingertips to massage tiny circles from the nape of your neck to your forehead, then across the hairline. For a once-or-twice weekly massage:

1. Brush your hair to remove contaminants and tangles.
2. Sit comfortably. Droop your head toward your chest and rotate it slowly to the right, then to the left.
3. Still leaning forward, place the palms of your hands (fingers separated) underneath your hair. Using push-and-relax movements, work your hands upward from the nape of your neck. Raise your head and reverse the process from forehead to nape. Repeat until your scalp feels tingly and warm.

Brushing: Why Gentle Is Better

Gentle brushing encourages blood circulation, stimulates the sebum-producing glands and distributes their oils to glimmerize hair strands. It also dislodges dry scalp flakes and whisks them away along with dust or hairspray residue. Brushing upward from the nape of the neck while bending forward adds volume after you flip it back into place. Overly vigorous brushing damages hair by stripping away outer cells to expose the inner shaft, breaking brittle hair, or by dislodging not-yet-ready-to-depart hairs.

How to Dry Clean Your Hair

These rub-in, brush-out cleansers can be utilized to remove surface soil, oil, and odor during illness or for any-time waterless freshening.

- *Almond meal, bran, cornmeal, oatmeal, sawdust* or *talc* can be sprinkled through the hair, massaged in for 5 minutes, then brushed out. Mixing a tablespoon of baking soda with any of these substances aids odor control.
- *Borax*, dissolved in alcohol and rubbed into well-brushed hair, then removed with a towel is a hundred-year-old solution.
- *Egg white*, beaten to a stiff meringue, rubbed into the hair and scalp and allowed to dry before being brushed out, is used for bedridden patients in European hospitals.
- *Witch hazel* or an antiseptic mouthwash, applied to the scalp and thoroughly brushed out, relieves "itchies" and removes surface contaminants. For blondes, 3 percent hydrogen peroxide will serve the same purpose and lighten hair roots.

How to Shampoo for Beautiful Hair

During the Middle Ages, shampooing bouffant coiffures was a semi-annual event. A century ago, ladies' magazines declared that hair could be washed as often as once a month. For your daily or weekly shampoo:

1. Rinse your hair with warm water.
2. Pour a little shampoo into your hands, then massage it into your scalp and hair. Always use as little shampoo as possible, and, if you are using a commercial product, dilute it with water.
3. Rinse with warm water until all the shampoo has gone down the drain. If your hair doesn't feel squeaky clean, apply a second lathering and repeat the rinsing.
4. Wrap a towel around your head; press to blot excess water, then dry gently.

Do-It-Yourself Shampoos That Clean and Enhance Your Hair

Body-cleansing bar soaps are not intended for hair. They can roughen the outer layer, dry the hair and scalp, and often contain chemicals that penetrate into the bloodstream through hair follicles. Alkaline hair products destroy the protective acid mantle and leave a film that, unless removed with an acidifying rinse, dulls hair and can create dandruff. You can improve commercial shampoos by adding a few drops of lemon juice to each application, or by combining equal amounts of shampoo and triple-strength herbal tea (camomile for light hair, rosemary or sage for dark). Or, you can concoct your own shampoo.

Castile shampoo

For shimmering blonde or silver hair, try this simple formula: Grate a 4-ounce bar of castile soap into a quart jar. Fill with water and let stand. Shake before using. Follow with a rinse of 2 tablespoons strained lemon juice in 3 cups water.

Herbal shampoos

For a cleansing, although not very sudsy, shampoo with an acceptable pH: Simmer 1/4 cup dried comfrey root or rosemary in 3 cups of water for 15 minutes. Strain, then add 1/2 cup grated castile soap and 1 teaspoon olive oil. Stir to dissolve the soap. For more lather, add 2 tablespoons of commercial shampoo.

Herbal extravaganza

5 cups water

1/4 cup *each* birch buds and leaves, marigold petals

1/4 cup dried orange peel from the spice shelf

2 tablespoons *each* camomile and red clover

1 tablespoon *each* orrisroot, nettle, rosemary, and sage

3/4 cup grated castile soap

2 tablespoons aloe vera gel

Bring water and herbs to boiling in a glass or enamel pan, cover and simmer for 15 minutes; steep for 30 minutes. Strain all but 1 cup of the liquid into a bowl with the soap, and beat until frothy. Whisk the remaining liquid with the aloe vera gel, then beat into the soapy mixture. For a sudsier shampoo, add 1/2 cup commercial shampoo.

Oil-enriched shampoos

To moisturize dry, brittle hair and add shine to normal hair, mix equal amounts of vegetable oil and your regular shampoo for the first lathering. Rinse thoroughly, then wash again with plain shampoo. For conditioning plus shine, add a few drops of jojoba or wheat germ oil or the contents of a 400-IU vitamin E capsule to enough of your regular shampoo for one lathering.

Protein shampoos

Shampoos with a protein content of 40 to 50 percent increase the tensile strength of hair, boost body, help repair dry hair, and add sheen. Commercial shampoos rarely contain more than 1 percent protein; you can improve them by adding natural protein.

- Soften half a packet of unflavored gelatin in 2 tablespoons cold water. Heat by placing the cup in a pan of boiling water or in a microwave oven for a few seconds, stir to dissolve, then add 1 tablespoon of mild shampoo.

- Whir 1 whole egg in an electric blender. Add 1 packet unflavored gelatin and 1/3 cup baby shampoo. Let stand for 5 minutes, then blend thoroughly. Or, whisk an egg with 2 tablespoons *each* water and your usual shampoo, plus 1 teaspoon *each* lemon juice and olive oil; reserve the surplus in the refrigerator. Or, whisk 1 egg yolk with the amount of shampoo you normally use.

- Separate an egg and beat the white. Mix in enough shampoo for two applications. Apply half the mixture, leave on for 5 minutes, then rinse. Massage the egg yolk into your scalp and hair; wait 5 minutes before rinsing with lukewarm water. Work in the remainder of the egg-white mixture and rinse thoroughly.

Sudsless shampoos

- *Alcohol and water.* Combine in the proportions of 1 part alcohol to 3 parts water.

- *Borax and sage tea or water.* Mix 2 tablespoons of borax with 1 quart of liquid.

- *Egg shampoos.* A whole egg or an egg yolk beaten with water is a soap-alternative for improving dry hair. For an "exemplary shampoo," the egg yolk can be beaten with rum.

Guidelines for Choosing a Hair Style
That Flatters Your Face

Upswept sides counterbalance gravity's sags, a double chin, or a short neck. A narrow jaw or receding chin can be modified by curls brought forward below the ears. A side part with soft curls framing the upper part of the face minimizes a prominent chin or a wide jawline. An oval face is compatible with all styles; hair-styling basics for other face shapes are

Diamond: bangs with volume at forehead, sleek sides, fullness at lower portion of face.

Heart: center or side part with wave across forehead, fullness at lower portion of face.

Long: bangs, width at sides, fluffed around the ears.

Round: sleek at sides with hair piled atop the head.

Square or rectangular: off-center part, bangs that sweep across forehead, sides drawn upward from ears to feathery curls on top.

How to Style as You Dry

Hair expands and loses its elasticity when wet. Vigorous rubbing with a towel, or stretching with a brush or a fine-toooothed comb, can break or dislodge waterlogged hair strands. Many hairstyles require only finger arranging and air drying; setting lotions coat each strand with a protective film for added body and style-holding.

Natural setting lotions, mousses, and gels

- **Beer,** allowed to stand until the carbonation dissipates, helps hold a set and control flyaway hair. Mix the beer half-and-half with water as a final rinse, or pour it into a spray bottle and mist your damp hair. Or, add 1 tablespoon of lemon juice to 1/3 cup of beer and comb it through your hair.
- **Egg white,** stiffly beaten, can be used as a protein-enriching styling mousse.

- **Flaxseed or quince seed.** Simmer 1 tablespoon of seeds in 1/2 cup water until slightly thickened. Strain before using.

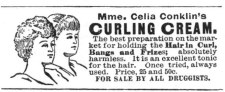
- **Gelatin.** Soften 1/2 packet unflavored gelatin in 2 tablespoons cold water. Add 1/3 cup boiling water, stir until dissolved, then blend in 1/2 teaspoon *each* lemon juice and cologne.

- **Lemon juice,** misted from a spray bottle and combed in, adds resiliency, body, and highlights to light hair.

- **Milk**—whole, for dry or normal hair; skim for oily hair—is an excellent wave set. For a gentle set, blend 1 teaspoon instant nonfat dry milk with 1/3 cup water.

- **Rosemary tea,** brewed double strength is a damp-weather curl preserver for dark hair.

Curling Cues

Always leave a bit of leeway between curlers and your scalp, and remove them as soon as your hair is dry. Thermostatically controlled hot rollers are considered safe, as are clips or plastic-tipped bobby pins. Heat from curling irons, crimpers, or hair dryers can be damaging if not carefully controlled. Back-combing or teasing is an unnatural way to style hair; the "body" it produces by roughing the cuticle can strip away the protective outer layer and lead to hair breakage.

Naturally Nurturing Hair Treatments

Eight preshampoo conditioners that are worth waiting for

Massage these natural conditioners into dry hair, cover with a shower cap and allow to permeate for 30 minutes to an hour before shampooing. To speed the penetration, wrap hot, moist towels around your head.

1. *Avocado* provides protein and oil for restoring rebellious hair to glossy manageability. Simply massage a mashed avocado into

your scalp and hair, or give your hair a super treat by blending the mashed avocado with a beaten egg and 2 tablespoons of wheat germ oil.

2. *Egg yolk* can be used as is, or, for dry hair, mixed with 2 teaspoons castor oil and 1 teaspoon rum. For an all-purpose conditioner: combine 1 egg yolk with 1/4 cup yogurt, 1 teaspoon grated lemon rind, and 1/2 teaspoon powdered kelp.

3. *Honey*. Light honey, all by its sticky self, does lovely things for light hair. For every shade of hair: mix 1/4 cup honey, 2 table-spoons vegetable oil, and 1 teaspoon lemon juice.

4. *Hydrolyzed protein* (predigested liquid protein marketed as a diet supplement) is a quickly absorbed substance for resurrecting life-less hair.

5. *Mayonnaise*, store bought or prepared from the recipe in the Glossary, is a mild conditioner. For additional body and glimmer, beat 1 egg yolk and 1 teaspoon *each* vinegar and powdered kelp into each application.

6. *Milk*. Mix instant nonfat dry milk and water to a paste for a body-building pack.

7. *Molasses* (light for light hair, dark for dark hair) is an old-fashioned favorite for rejuvenating weary hair. Soften 1 packet unflavored gelatin in 2 tablespoons molasses. Stir in 1 tablespoon *each* flat beer and sweetened condensed milk.

8. *Oils*. Polyunsaturated oils combat dryness and revitalize drab, brittle hair. Warm the oil to room temperature if it has been refrigerated; shampoo twice for total removal. For extra shine and easier removal, mix 2 tablespoons oil with 1 tablespoon lemon juice and 1 teaspoon cognac. Castor oil strengthens hair weakened by overprocessing or overexposure to sun and water. Linseed oil (from a health food outlet, not a paint store) softens stiff, unman-ageable hair.

After-shampoo quicker-acting conditioners

Conditioners such as these should be applied only to the hair, not the scalp. To use: Pour the conditioner into your hands, rub into your freshly shampooed hair, comb through for even distribution, then rinse out with tepid water after the suggested length of time. To add sheen, blend 1 tablespoon citric acid crystals with any of these conditioners. For extra body plus shine, follow any of them with a 3-minute application of mayonnaise.

- *Eggs.* Beat 1 or 2 egg yolks with 1 or 2 tablespoons of water (depending on hair length), rinse after 15 minutes. To increase the benefits, blend 2 tablespoon yogurt with each egg yolk. A whole egg can be whisked with lemon juice for a 15-minute conditioning shiner-upper, or gussied up for other head-mending nourishers.

  Combine 1 beaten egg with 1 tablespoon *each* glycerin and wheat germ oil. Or, dissolve 1 tablespoon citric acid crystals in 2 tablespoons water, then beat in 1 egg and 1 tablespoon sweetened condensed milk.

- *Fruit salad.* In an electric blender, whir 1/2 a banana, 1/4 of an avocado, 1/6 of a cantaloupe, and 1 tablespoon *each* wheat germ oil and yogurt. Leave on for 10 minutes to regenerate summer-abused hair.

- *Half-and-Half* gives hair extra body when left on for 5 minutes.

Conditioning with rinses

Adding a tablespoon of lemon juice (for light hair) or cider vinegar (for dark hair) to a quart of water for the final rinse removes dulling film and restores the pH balance. (Strain the juice through a sieve. If you rely on the juicer strainer you may think you've developed a terminal scalp disease when fragments of lemon pulp appear in your hair.)

- **Baking soda,** mixed with water in the proportions of 1 tablespoon soda to 3/4 cup water, will remove hairspray residue and discourage unpleasant odor. Work the liquid through your hair, then rinse out.

- **Herbal teas** (camomile for blondes, rosemary or sage for brunettes) brewed regular strength and used for a final rinse, tone the hair and restore the acid mantle.

- **Vinegar.** Combine 2 tablespoons *each* vinegar and double-strength peppermint tea with 1 quart of water as a final rinse. To liven drab hair, mix 1/4 cup vinegar with 1-1/4 cups water; dispel the odor by adding a few drops of oil of cloves to a pint of water and rinsing again.

  Cosmetic vinegars have a more pleasing aroma plus increased conditioning benefits. Two tablespoons of any of the cosmetic vinegars in Chapter 3 may be added to your final rinse, or you can brew your own customized rinse. Each combination should be brought to a boil in an enamel or glass pan and simmered, uncovered, for 15 minutes, then covered and allowed to steep for 30 minutes before straining.

All-purpose sparkler

1 cup *each* white vinegar and distilled water
1/4 cup *each* dried nettle, red clover, and rosemary

Light-haired vinegar rinse

1 cup *each* white vinegar and distilled water
3 camomile tea bags
2 tablespoons lemon juice

Dark-haired sage rinse

1 cup *each* red wine vinegar and distilled water
2 tablespoons dried sage

Conditioning with tonics and dressings

Tonics may be applied between shampoos or immediately after shampooing to condition, control, and add shine. You can substitute 80-proof vodka for the ethyl alcohol in any of these preparations.

- **Castor oil**, totally soluble in alcohol, has an advantage over other oils for hair dressings. For an instant tonic, shake 1/4 cup water with 2 tablespoons ethyl alcohol and 2 teaspoons *each* castor oil, ammonia, and glycerin.

  Antiseptic tonics. Steep 2 tablespoons *each* nettle and sage in 1-1/2 cups ethyl alcohol for a week. Strain out the herbs, pour the liquid into a pint bottle, add 1/3 cup castor oil, and shake well. Or, steep 1/4 cup sage , 2 tablespoons rosemary, and 1 table-spoon nettle in 1-1/2 cups ethyl alcohol for 10 days. Strain; then add 1/4 cup distilled water and 1/4 cup castor oil. Shake to combine.

- **Perfumed tonic.** This exotic blend originated in Arab harems and is said to stimulate hair growth as well as furnish fragrance and shine. Add 2 tablespoons lavender water and 1/2 teaspoon *each* lavender oil and sweet basil oil to 1 pint ethyl alcohol. Let stand for a month, shaking every few days.

- **Rose water and glycerin.** Mix half-and-half or in a ratio of 3 parts rose water to 1 part glycerin.

How to Enliven Your Hair Color
with Natural Colorants

Hair pigmentation is not necessarily permanent. Tow-headed children often become brunette adults, carrot-tops may turn into auburn-haired sirens or sires, and we all eventually grow gray. If your present hair color is less than exciting, natural substances can add pizazz. Vegetable hair dyes date back to antiquity; walnut hulls and henna are two naturally conditioning colorants currently available.

BLACK WALNUT. The hulls of black walnuts (sold in health food stores) can be pressed to produce a juice that dyes hair dark brown. It also stains skin; wear rubber gloves when handling the hulls, and apply dye carefully. For a rich walnut hue: Combine 1/4 cup walnut juice, 1 tablespoon ethyl alcohol, and 1/4 teaspoon *each* ground cinnamon and cloves in a screw-top jar. Let stand for a week, shaking daily, then strain through a cloth lined sieve and add 1/8 teaspoon salt.

HENNA. Today's henna is more sophisticated than the stewed henna-bush leaves used thousands of years ago by Persian and Egyptian beauties to color their hair and nails. Dried and powdered, henna is marketed in neutral, black, and brown, as well as red shades. It coats the hair to add body and color, then gradually fades away without leaving an obvious root line. Intensity varies with the length of application and henna is not recommended if your hair is more than 15 percent gray, if it has been bleached or colored with a metallic dye, or if you plan to have a perm in the immediate future.

How to brighten dark hair

Camomile tea, brewed regular-strength, brightens dark hair without bleaching it. Rosemary and sage teas (individually or combined and steeped double strength) darken while they add glimmer. Leave the tea on your hair for half an hour, then rinse with warm water.

How to liven light hair

- **Camomile** brightens blonde hair, minimizes dark streaks, adds highlights, and abolishes the spongy stickiness that can occur with bleached hair. As a final rinse, pour regular or double-strength camomile tea through your hair several times. For additional glimmer, add 1 teaspoon lemon juice. For more bleaching action, brew triple-strength camomile tea with white wine instead of water.

- **Green pekoe tea**, brewed regular strength and used as a final rinse adds a reddish shimmer to blonde or light brown hair.

  Cindy's strawberry-blonde hair had gradually faded to such a nondescript shade that she threatened to have it tinted before leaving for college. As an alternative, Cindy's grandmother suggested she try tea. "Worked wonders for me," she said. "My hair used to be reddish-gold, and when I was 19, my aunt accused me of coloring it. I told her honestly, 'All I do is wash and rinse it.' I just didn't mention that the rinse was green pekoe!" The tea's magic was as effective as it had been 50 years earlier; red glints illuminated Cindy's bright "untinted" hair as she boarded the plane for school.

- **Lemon** brings sunny glints to light hair. Combine 1/2 cup water with 1/3 cup strained lemon juice. Work through the hair, then let dry before rinsing.

  Lemon-lime shampoo. Combine 1 tablespoon *each* lemon juice, lime juice, and a mild shampoo. Work through your dry hair with fingers or a wide-toothed comb. Dry with a blow dryer or sit in the sun for 20 minutes. Wash out and follow with a rinse of 1 tablespoon lemon juice per pint of water. Repeat daily until the desired shade is achieved.

  Lemon hair spray. To combine brightening with style holding, mist with lemon juice. For more holding power, simmer a cut-up lemon in water to cover. When the lemon is tender, pour the mixture into an electric blender. Whir until smooth, then strain through a fine sieve.

- **Peroxide** brightens murky looking light hair, but is not recommended for tinted or bleached hair. Combine 2 tablespoons peroxide with 1 tablespoon mild shampoo and 1/8 teaspoon ammonia. Work through wet hair and leave on for 4 minutes. Rinse out, then rewash with plain shampoo and follow with a lemon-water rinse. For a more pronounced effect, use 20-volume peroxide instead of 10-volume.

- **Natural frosting.** Fresh lemon juice, camomile oil, peroxide, or the lemon-lime shampoo described above, can be used to frost light brown or dark blonde hair. Use a small brush to "paint" random strands; or don a "frosting cap" (or a punctured bathing cap), pull the strands through with a crochet hook and saturate with a cotton ball. Sit in the sun a few minutes before shampooing.

How to Postpone and Rejuvenate Gray Hair

Illness may cause alternating bands of gray on each hair as pigment-forming capability fluctuates with the severity of the disease. Normal graying commences around the age of forty; premature graying is linked to heredity, stress, and nutritional deficiencies. Stress management and dietary upgrading often forestall and sometimes regress the silvering; color is not restored to already-white hairs but their replacements grow out in the original shade. Nutritionists report astounding successes with several months of a high-protein diet plus two tablespoons each of brewers yeast and vegetable oil daily, and these anti-gray-hair vitamins: 1 B-complex stress tab, 30 to 300 milligrams B-5, 2,000 milligrams choline, 400 to 800 micrograms folic acid, and 100 to 300 milligrams PABA. Nineteenth-century suggestions include these gray-hair preventives and restoratives:

- Blend 2 tablespoons castor oil and 1 tablespoon ethyl alcohol, Rub into hair roots once each week.

- Combine 2 tablespoons *each* glycerin and rose water or cologne with 1 tablespoon cider vinegar. Each morning and evening, brush your hair until your scalp tingles, then apply the liquid to the hair roots with a cotton ball.

- Drink a cup of sage tea daily and rub a bit of the brew onto the hair roots. Or, simmer 1 tablespoon *each* black pekoe tea and dried sage in 1 cup water in a covered pan for 20 minutes. Steep several hours before straining. Massage the liquid into your hair and scalp each day until hair is the desired shade, then reduce applications to twice weekly.

How to Correct Seven Specific Hair and Scalp Problems

1. Dandruff and itchy scalp

That little itch and the snow descending upon your shoulders may be only dry flakes from hairspray residue or shampoo buildup. Daily brushing plus frequent shampooing preceded by an oil-based conditioner and followed with an acidic rinse may be all that is required. Dandruff that persists may be the real thing, *seborrheic dermatitis*, which can develop when the sebaceous glands are overactive as a result of emotional tension or faulty diet, or can appear as a byproduct of allergy, hormonal imbalance, or infection. Studies show that many cases of dandruff are related to poor metabolization of refined carbohydrates and the resulting deficiency of B vitamins. Improving your diet and taking antioxidants (30 to 400 IU vitamin E plus 50 to 200 micrograms selenium daily) may help correct the cause. Immediate control often can be achieved with these natural precautions and remedies:

- Massage your scalp daily with castor oil or olive oil; castor oil mixed half-and-half with vinegar; vinegar or lemon juice diluted with an equal amount of water or mint tea; any of the cosmetic vinegars from Chapter 3; a mixture of 1 tablespoon glycerin and 1 teaspoon cider vinegar, or 1 teaspoon *each* glycerin and borax blended with 1/4 cup distilled water; double-strength mint tea or rosemary-sage tea with 1 teaspoon borax dissolved in each cup; rubbing alcohol or witch hazel.

- Between shampoos, work cornmeal or miller's bran through your hair and brush out.

- Before shampooing, rub petroleum jelly or olive oil into your scalp and cover with a hot, moist towel for 30 minutes. Or, massage a lightly beaten egg (with or without a tablespoon of sea salt) into your dry hair and scalp. Let it permeate for 5 minutes before rinsing and shampooing. If your hair is dry, use egg yolks instead of a whole egg. If your hair is oily but your scalp is dry, substitute egg white beaten with the juice of a lemon.

- Follow each shampoo with a final rinse of strong tea: catnip, celery-seed, rosemary-mint, or wintergreen; add 1 tablespoon vinegar to increase the benefits. After the rinse, massage your scalp with a mixture of 1/4 cup apple cider vinegar, 1 tablespoon witch hazel, and 2 crushed aspirins.

- Always dry your hair with fresh towels, and always use your own combs and hairbrushes; infectious bacteria is transferable.

2. Dry hair

The amount of sebum produced by the sebaceous glands diminishes with age and is responsible for gradually drying hair. Adding 2 tablespoons of vegetable oil plus vitamin E and cod liver oil supplements to the daily diet, brushing nightly, having occasional preshampoo oil treatments, and shampooing no more often than twice a week usually corrects this type of dryness.

Suddenly dry, lifeless, brittle hair can occur during periods of stress, pregnancy, or illness; or can be brought about by overprocessing or overexposure to extreme temperatures. Vitamin-C deficiency inhibits the oil-producing glands and may cause hair to split or break. To revitalize your forlorn tresses, pamper them with natural nurturing.

- Brush your hair gently to avoid breakage while distributing the natural oils.
- Use a preshampoo protein/oil conditioner each time you wash your hair. Extend the length of conditioner contact time or drape a heating pad set on "low" over your conditioning hair for 30 minutes.
- Enrich your shampoo with oil or protein, and use a mildly acidic solution such as 1 teaspoon lemon juice or vinegar per pint of water for the final rinse.

3. Oily hair

Reducing dietary fats and experimenting with these natural remedies should bring liveliness to your lank locks.

- Work a strip of gauze through your hairbrush bristles to absorb excess oil during your daily brushing.
- Before you shampoo, apply stiffly beaten egg white to your hair and scalp, then brush out after it dries. Or, dissolve 1 tablespoon salt in skim milk and rub it into your scalp. Shampoo after 30 minutes.
- Follow each shampoo with a rinse of 1 tablespoon lemon juice or vinegar per pint of water.
- Before styling your hair, rub witch hazel on your scalp.

4. Split ends

Split ends are often a corollary of dry hair; especially when it has been overpermed, set with brush rollers, or teased while styling. Singeing split ends is not recommended (it can harm the hair shafts); trimming them off prevents the separation of cell layers from extending throughout the length of the hair. Dry-hair care, plus refraining from further hair-wrecking practices, should avoid recurrence of the problem.

5. Fallout and thinning hair

The diameter of each hair and their total number varies with hair color; blondes have more but skinnier hair than brunettes or redheads.

As metabolic processes slow, Father Time gradually makes fat hair thin, thick hair sparse. Females are less prone to baldness than males, but our equalization of rights is rapidly equalizing hair fallout as well as pay scales because of the accompanying stress that constricts follicle openings and nourishment-carrying blood vessels. Anything that disrupts our internal system contributes to hair loss: malnutrition, pregnancy, severe illness, an underactive thyroid, certain medications, chemical or X-ray therapy.

Nutritional deficiencies or an excess of carbohydrates and animal fats can cause falling hair. Increasing protein intake by 14 grams a day (the amount in 2 eggs or 1-1/2 cups skim milk) increases the diameter of each hair by 14 percent;[80] B-vitamin-containing foods (see Vitamin and Mineral Chart) stimulate hair growth. To augment the daily diet, nutritionists suggest 1 multivitamin-mineral, 1 B-complex stress tab, 1,000 milligrams *each* choline and inositol, and 1,000 milligrams of vitamin C.

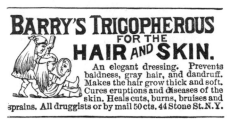

External care is also important. About 85 percent of our hair is normally in its growing phase; the hairs that fall are those that have loosened in the follicles to make way for their replacements. Overly enthusiastic brushing or toweling can prematurely dislodge these hairs, or break them off in the follicles to prevent or slow the emergence of new hair. Accumulations of dead cells, dirt, or shampoo residue can hamper regrowth by clogging the tiny openings. Consistently gentle cleanliness and these natural growth encouragers often resolve the problem.

- Two or three times a day, massage a small amount of one of these old-fashioned ointments into your scalp: a blend of 2 tablespoons *each* castor oil and lard with 1/4 teaspoon rosemary oil. Or, 1/4 cup almond oil or olive oil with 1/2 teaspoon rosemary oil and 3 drops lemon-grass oil.
- Twice daily, massage your scalp and hairline in small circular motions with your fingertips or an electric vibrator, preferably while relaxing on a slantboard with your head 18 inches lower than your feet.

Or, stimulate circulation with this 1850s cure for falling hair. Immerse your head in cold water containing 1 tablespoon salt per quart. Dry your hair, then brush until your scalp feels warm.

- At bedtime, try one of these natural remedies: massage your scalp with aloe vera gel, sliced raw garlic, jojoba oil, lard, or fresh onion juice. Shampoo out in the morning. To augment the benefits, rub petroleum jelly into your freshly scrubbed scalp and wipe it off with cotton saturated in a mixture of 1/4 cup water and 1 teaspoon alcohol.

- Once each week, apply a preshampoo protein or oil conditioner, or a 2-hour preshampoo scalp-stimulator of 2 tablespoons vodka mixed with 1 tablespoon honey. Then use a protein-enriched, body-building shampoo.

- Use rosemary tea as an after-shampoo rinse. Or, cook 1/4 pound of unpeeled chopped chestnuts in 1 quart of boiling water for 10 minutes. Cover and let stand for 15 minutes. Strain and add 1 teaspoon wine vinegar. Pour 1 cupful through your hair as a final rinse.

6. Localized loss

Any of the falling-hair instigators may be responsible for a receding hairline or patchy bald spots, but hair styling is the customary culprit. Men are burdened with MPB (male pattern baldness) genes; women denude their own scalps. *Alopecia areata* or *traction alopecia* is the technical term for what happens when we roll our hair too tightly or try to sleep on brush rollers, pull it back into a sleek chignon style, plait it into cornrows, or strangle it with rubber bands for a pony tail. Although prolonged tension can cause permanent hair loss,[149] hair usually regrows when the abusive practices are discontinued.

7. Swimmer's hair

Ocean salt, lake minerals, or the algicides and chlorine in swimming pools strip away the hair's protective covering and oils, and can turn blonde, gray, or bleached hair an eerie shade of green. To avoid these misfortunes: wear a bathing cap lined around the hairline with a 2-inch strip of chamois. Immediately after emerging, rinse your hair with fresh water or spray it with bottled water, club soda, or a solution of baking soda and water; then shampoo as soon as possible.

Judy didn't think she needed to wear a bathing cap while swimming her daily laps because she kept her head out of the water. After a few weeks, however, the sides and back of her bright golden hair acquired the greenish cast of aging copper. When shampooing failed to remove the discoloration, Judy sought professional help. "Tomato juice works better than anything," said the salon manager. "If that doesn't get rid of the green, come in for a hot-oil pack and chemical treatment." Judy applied an oil treatment at home, left the tomato juice on her hair for 5 minutes after shampooing, and was rewarded with a return to her standard gold. To prevent future greening, Judy rinses her hair with tomato juice whenever the edges of her hair feel damp after swimming.

Lifetime Beauty & Health: Diet, Exercise, & Stress Management

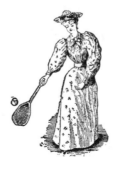

❧ 15 ❧

How to Eat Your Way to Beauty & Health: The Basics of Balancing Your Diet

Your glowing complexion, strong nails, sparkling eyes, shining hair, and vibrantly healthy body reflect the nourishment they receive from the foods you eat. Balancing a diet can be as simple as selecting servings from the four basic food groups categorized in the U.S. Department of Agriculture's nutritional guidelines.

Appetizing Comestibles from the Four Basic Food Groups

1. Fruits and Vegetables

Eating a variety of fruits and vegetables provides vitamins, minerals, fiber, and complex carbohydrates. The recommended daily minimum is one serving of fruit, one of a dark-green or dark-yellow vegetable, one of a starchy root vegetable, and one of raw vegetables. Serving size is

1 whole fruit such as an apple, banana, or orange

1/2 cantaloupe or grapefruit

1/2 cup sliced raw or cooked fruit or berries

3/4 cup fruit or vegetable juice

1/2 cup chopped raw or cooked vegetable

1 medium-size potato

1 small salad

Variety is essential because no one food contains the full spectrum of necessary nutrients. To preserve their maximum benefits, subject vegetables to a minimum of preparation. Never soak them in water or add baking soda to enhance color while cooking, and cook in as little water as possible unless the liquid is to be consumed in soups. Store all leftovers lightly covered; orange juice, for instance, loses 15 percent of its vitamin C if refrigerated for a day in an open pitcher.

Dietary fiber (the indigestible portion of plant foods) is divided into two categories:

- **Soluble fiber** (pectins and gums from fruits, nuts, oats, seeds, vegetables) helps the body metabolize carbohydrates and reduce cholesterol.

- **Insoluble fiber** (cellulose, lignin, and hemicellulose from whole grains) helps prevent constipation, diverticulosis, and colon cancer.

The National Cancer Institute recommends a daily mixture of 25 to 30 grams of "soluble" and "insoluble"; both categories are charted under the single heading, "fiber" in Table 15-1.

2. Breads, cereals, and other grains

Cereals and grains are our principal source of fiber (see Table 15-2), furnish a wealth of vitamins and minerals, and, when combined with legumes or milk, provide complete protein with less fat than meat. Official guidelines recommend that at least one of the four daily servings from this food group be of a cereal; one of a whole-grain product.

1 slice of bread or 1 muffin, roll, or tortilla

1/2 to 3/4 cup cooked cereal, pasta, or rice

1/2 to 1 cup (depending on density) ready-to-eat cereal

TABLE 15-1: FRUIT AND VEGETABLE FOOD COMPOSITION*

per serving	Vit A IU	Vit C mg	Fiber grams	Carbohydrate grams	Calories
Apple, fresh	117	5	2.4	17	76
Asparagus; cut, cooked	866	25	1.7	3	20
Banana, raw	285	15	2.7	30	128
Broccoli; fresh, cut	2,580	108	3.9	5	30
Cabbage; raw, shredded	60	25	3.4	3	12
Carrots; raw, grated	11,000	8	3.3	10	42
Corn, vacuum canned	320	5	4.0	33	105
Orange, fresh	360	90	2.0	20	88
Peach, fresh	1,516	8	2.3	10	43
Peas; frozen, cooked	480	11	3.2	10	55
Potato, baked white	—	20	1.0	21	93
Strawberries, sliced	60	60	1.8	9	40
Tomato, raw	1,100	28	1.4	6	25

*Varies with growth and preparation methods. Figures complied from *Eat Better, Live Better*,[63] *Nutrition Almanac*,[86] and *U.S.D.A. Handbook No. 8.*

TABLE 15-2: FOOD COMPOSITION OF GRAIN PRODUCTS*

per serving	Carbohy-drate grams	Protein grams	Fat grams	Fiber grams	Calories
Breads—1 slice					
Cornbread	14	3.7	3.6	1.9	104
Pumpernickel	17	3.0	.4	1.5	79
White	12	2.0	.7	.7	62
Whole-wheat	11	3.0	.6	1.3	55
Cereals					
Cornflakes (1 cup)	21	2.0	.1	4.1	95
Oats, cooked (3/4 cup)	18	4.8	1.7	3.6	103
Shredded wheat (1 large biscuit)	20	2.0	1.0	3.3	90
Crackers					
Graham (2 crack-ers)	10	1.0	1.0	1.4	55
Saltines (4 crackers)	8	1.0	1.0	.1	50
Rice—1/2 cup					
Brown, cooked	17	1.9	.4	1.8	89
White, cooked	18	1.5	.1	.6	80

*Compiled from: *Eat Better, Live Better,*63 *Nutrition Almanac,*86 and *U.S.D.A. Handbook No. 8.*

3. Milk and milk products

When the body is deprived of an adequate supply of calcium it draws this mineral from our bony structure to maintain the soft tissues and nervous system, and leaves us with porous bones and loose teeth. The minimum requirement of two cups of milk (or the equivalent in milk products) provides over two thirds of the RDA for calcium, almost a fourth of our daily protein, plus carbohydrates for energy (see Table 15-3), and, if the milk has been fortified, one third of the RDA for vitamins A and D. Skim and reduced-fat milk products furnish the benefits without all the saturated fat of whole milk. You can select your quota from these serving-size guidelines:

> 1 cup fluid milk, reconstituted dry milk, or plain yogurt
>
> 1/2 cup cottage cheese (calcium equals 1/4 cup milk)
>
> 1/2 cup ice cream (calcium equals 1/3 cup milk)
>
> 1-inch cube Cheddar or Swiss cheese (calcium equals 3/4 cup milk)
>
> 2 tablespoons processed cheese spread (calcium equals 1/2 cup milk)

4. Meat, fish, poultry, eggs, legumes, and nuts

Protein from this food group should be ingested daily to maintain beautiful externals such as hair and nails, and vital internals such as muscles and organs. Meat and dairy products are complete- protein foods. Plant foods, with the exception of soybeans, must have their missing amino acids supplied by combining them with other protein sources. Two daily servings are all that are required, and the serving-size is surprisingly small, as shown in Table 15-4. The protein equivalents for 1 ounce of cooked meat are

> 1 egg
>
> 1/2 to 3/4 cup cooked legumes
>
> 1/4 to 1/2 cup nuts or seeds
>
> 2 tablespoons peanut butter

TABLE 15-3: FOOD COMPOSITION OF MILK AND MILK PRODUCTS*

per serving	Cal-cium	Protein grams	Fat grams	Carbo-hy-drate grams	Calo-ries
Milk					
1 cup whole	291	8.0	8.1	11.0	150
2 percent	297	8.0	5.0	12.0	120
skim	302	8.0	trace	12.0	85
buttermilk	285	8.0	2.0	12.0	100
Evaporated milk (1/2 cup)	328	8.5	9.5	12.5	170
Cream, whipped (2 tablespoons)	10	trace	6.0	trace	80
Sour cream (2 tablespoons)	28	trace	2.0	2.0	50
Ice cream (1/2 cup)	88	2.5	7.0	16.0	135
Ice milk (1/2 cup)	88	2.5	3.0	14.0	92
Yogurt					
1 cup whole milk	274	8.0	7.0	11.0	140
nonfat plus added milk solids	452	13.0	trace	17.0	125
Cottage cheese					
1/2 cup large curd, creamed	68	14.0	5.0	3.0	117
low-fat, 2 percent	78	15.5	2.0	4.0	102
Cheddar cheese, 1-inch cube	204	7.0	9.0	trace	115
Swiss cheese, 1-inch cube	272	8.0	8.0	1.0	105
Parmesan cheese, grated (2 tablespoons)	69	2.0	2.0	trace	25

*Compiled from *Eat Better, Live Better,*[63] *Nutrition Almanac,*[86] and *U.S.D.A. Handbook No. 8.*

TABLE 15-4: FOOD COMPOSITION OF MEAT, FISH, POULTY, EGGS, LEGUMES, AND NUTS*

per serving (meats measured after cooking)	Protein grams	Fat grams	Carbohydrate grams	Calories
Beef—lean				
steak; broiled (2 X 4 X 1/2 inch)	18	4	0	115
ground; broiled (3-1/2-inch patty)	23	10	0	185
Fish				
nonoily, baked (3 ounces)	22	4	0	135
tuna; oil pack, drained (3 ounces)	24	7	0	170
Chicken, 1/2 breast, fried in oil	26	5	1	160
Turkey—roasted				
dark meat (3 ounces)	26	7	0	175
light meat (3 ounces)	28	3	0	150
Egg; 1 large, boiled	6	6	trace	80
Legumes—dry; cooked, drained (1/2 cups)				
black-eyed peas	6	trace	17	80
lima	8	trace	25	130
red or white	8	trace	21	115
soybeans (complete protein)	11	6	11	130
Nuts—1/4 cup				
Cashews	6	16	10	199
Pecans, broken	3	17	4	160
Walnuts, chopped	4	16	4	161
Peanut butter (2 tablespoons)	8	16	6	180
Sunflower seeds; hulled (1/4 cup)	9	15	7	178

*Compiled from *Eat Better, Live Better*,63 *Nutrition Almanac*,86 and *U.S.D.A. Handbook No. 8.*

How to Eat by the Numbers

For a more exactingly balanced diet you can divide foods into three categories (carbohydrates, fats, proteins) and work with percentages. The National Institutes of Health recommends that the diet for a moderately active adult consist of 55 to 60 percent carbohydrate, 25 to 30 percent fat, and no more than 15 percent protein.[170] Being precise requires an elaborate set of charts, but you can approximate with the food-composition information in this chapter.

- One gram equals 1/28 of an ounce; 100 grams (3-1/2 ounces) equal approximately 1/2 cup of juices and foods such as cooked vegetables. One milligram equals 1/1000 of a gram; a microgram is 1/1000 of a milligram.

- A calorie is a measure of the amount of energy produced when a food is "burned" by the body. Excess calories are stored as body fat. Caloric needs can be estimated by multiplying your ideal weight by 15. For instance, if you weigh 125 pounds, 1,875 calories a day should maintain your weight.

Carbohydrates, at 57 percent of the 1,875 calories, equal 1069 calories or 267 grams.

Fat's 30 percent proportion equals 562 calories or 62 grams.

Protein, computed at 13 percent, equals 243 calories or 61 grams for a 125-pound individual.

CONVERSION FORMULA

Carbohydrates	4 calories per gram	112 calories per ounce
Fats	9 calories per gram	252 calories per ounce
Proteins	4 calories per gram	112 calories per ounce

Carbohydrates

Complex carbohydrates from the starches and fibers of plant foods are the hi-octane fuel that furnishes energy most efficiently. Simple carbohydrates include the glucose and fructose from fruits and vegetables, lactose from milk, and sucrose from cane sugar. Fructose is gradually assimilated because of the accompanying fiber. Candy or sugary desserts, especially when eaten alone, immediately raise the blood sugar level, provide a brief spurt of energy, then leave us with the wearies because the insulin released to cope with the sudden surge of glucose also disposes of sugar that was already in the blood. Molasses, honey, and brown sugar contain minuscule amounts of vitamins and minerals, but from a nutritional standpoint, sweets are unnecessary; the body readily converts complex carbohydrates into glucose for our energy needs. As long as most of your carbohydrate quota is supplied by vegetables, fruits, grains, and legumes (and you are neither diabetic nor hypoglycemic), occasionally indulging a chocaholic craving or a yen for lemon meringue should not unduly upset your dietary balance.

Table 15-5 shows the caloric breakdown of bakery products and desserts.

TABLE 15-5: FOOD COMPOSITION OF BAKERY PRODUCTS AND DESSERTS*

per serving	Carbohydrate grams	Protein grams	Fat grams	Calories
Cake				
Angel food	24.0	2.8	.1	108
Devil's food cupcake with chocolate frosting	28.0	2.1	8.2	184
White, 2-layer with white frosting	94.2	5.0	19.3	562
Candy				
Chocolate fudge (1-inch piece)	34.0	1.2	5.5	180
Marshmallow (2 large)	9.4	.2	trace	38
Cookies—1 average				
Brownie with nuts	25.0	3.3	16.0	243
Chocolate chip	6.0	.5	3.0	52
Fig bar	11.5	.6	.9	55
Danish pastry, without nuts	30.0	4.8	15.2	274
Doughnuts—1 average Cake	17.0	1.5	6.1	129
Raised, jelly filled	30.0	3.4	8.8	226
Pie—1/6 of 9-inch pie				
Apple	59.9	3.5	17.4	402
Lemon meringue	52.7	5.2	14.3	356
Pecan	70.5	7.0	31.5	574
Pumpkin	37.1	6.0	17.0	319

*Compiled from *The Dieter's Companion*,66 *Nutrition Almanac*,86 and *USDA Handbook No. 8.*

Fats and oils

Without at least one tablespoon of fat every day, fat-soluble nutrients are not assimilated, hair is lackluster, skin flakes, and joints creak. The fatty acids from unsaturated fats are termed "essential" because they cannot be produced from other fats within the body. Fats from plant products (except for coconut or palm oil) are unsaturated and remain liquid at room temperature; animal fats are saturated, contain cholesterol, and harden at room temperature. Hydrogenated vegetable fats have been converted to a solid form that, according to reports in *Prevention* (June 1988), may be more harmful than naturally saturated fats. Michael E. DeBakey,[51] has found that cholesterol levels are not affected by an occasional steak or a few eggs each week. (See Table 15-6.)

TABLE 15-6: FOOD COMPOSITION OF FATS AND OILS*

per table-spoon	Total Fat grams	Fatty Acids Saturated grams	Unsaturated Oleic/Linolic grams	Choles-terol mg	Calories
Butter	11.8	7.2	3.2	30	100
Margarine					
regular	11.8	2.1	8.4	0	100
whipped	8.0	1.4	5.7	0	70
Lard	12.8	5.1	6.4	12	116
Vegetable shortening	12.0	3.2	8.8	0	110
Oils					
corn	13.6	1.7	11.1	0	120
olive	13.5	1.9	10.8	0	119
peanut	13.5	2.3	10.4	0	119
safflower	13.6	1.0	11.6	0	120
Mayonnaise	11.0	2.0	8.0	5	100
Salad dressing					
French	6.0	1.1	4.5	0	65
Italian	9.0	1.6	6.6	0	70

*Varies among different brands. Compiled from *The Dieter's Companion*,[66] *Eat Better, Live Better*,[63] and *Jane Brody's Nutrition Book*.[28]

Proteins

For complete proteins, combine foods such as cereal and milk, bread and peanut butter or cheese, or beans and rice; or utilize the already-complete proteins from animal products. All foods (except fats and sugars contain some protein). A pint of milk provides 16 grams of protein, two slices of wheat bread furnish 6 grams; filling out the 61-gram quota (267 calories) for a 125- pound person presents no problem. The trick lies in keeping fat and cholesterol within sensible limits.

Only about 15 percent of our cholesterol is acquired from foods; the remainder is manufactured by the body to help produce new cells and to keep the brain and nervous system functioning. There are two kinds of cholesterol: the damaging, low-density liptoproteins (LDL) which cling to arterial walls; and the protective, high-density liptoproteins (HDL) which help the body eliminate excess cholesterol.

Eggs, the most perfect protein, have their yolks loaded with cholesterol, yet contain lecithin (a phospholipid that helps regulate cholesterol), and, according to a report in *Nutrition Action Health Letter* (July/August 1989), each egg now contains 22 percent less cholesterol than the "official" measurement of 274 milligrams shown in Table 15-7. Shellfish are so low in saturated fat that their cholesterol content is not considered nearly as health-threatening as the lesser amounts from highly saturated sources such as red meat; whose fat and cholesterol is also being reduced by dietary improvements.

Condiments and Seasonings

Apparently insignificant extras can wreak havoc with a perfectly balanced diet. (See Table 15-8.)

Salt/Sodium

Whether provided by Mother Nature or added to foods as table salt, sodium is vital for physical and mental health. Without salt we become apathetic or our muscles cramp; with an overabundance, our skin puffs and our bloodpressure soars. Fewer than 30 percent of us are born with the genetic predisposition to hypertension that requires severe sodium limitation, but most of us use too much salt. The suggested maximum is 2,500 milligrams daily; the current average is 4,845 milligrams.[168] Dr. Richard Moore, co-author of *The K Factor* (Macmillan Publishing, 1986), has found that maintaining an equal balance of potassium with sodium can prevent many salt-instigated problems. Salt substitutes have most of their sodium replaced by potassium but they should be used only with medical approval—a potassium overload can be equally hazardous to your health. Herbs and spices safely enhance flavors without adding sodium.

TABLE 15-7: FOOD COMPOSITION OF PROTEINS*

protein source	Protein grams	Fatty Acids		Choles- terol mg	Calories
		Satu- rated grams	Unsaturated Oleic/Linolic grams		
Beef; lean, cooked, 3 ounces	26	2.7	2.7	80	172
Cheese—1-inch cube					
Cheddar	7	6.1	2.3	30	115
Mozzarella	8	4.4	1.7	25	90
Cream cheese, 1 ounce	2	6.2	2.6	30	100
Chicken, broiled, 3 ounces	21	1.1	1.9	60	120
Egg—1 large					
Whole, boiled	6	1.7	2.6	274	80
White only	3	0	0	0	15
Yolk only	3	1.7	2.6	274	65
Fish—3 ounces					
Haddock; breaded, fried	17	1.4	3.3	60	140
Shrimp; canned, drained	21	.1	.2	113	100
Tuna; water pack, drained	24	1.5	2.2	48	105
Frankfurter; 1, 2 ounces	7	5.6	7.7	35	170
Milk—1 cup					
Whole	8	5.1	2.3	35	150
1 percent	8	1.6	.8	8	100
Yogurt; low-fat 1 cup	13	.3	.1	12	125

*Varies with product and preparation. Compiled from *The Dieter's Companion*[66] *Eat Better, Live Better*,[63] and *Jane Brody's Nutrition Book*.[28]

TABLE 15-8: FOOD COMPOSITION OF CONDIMENTS AND SEA-SONINGS*

per amount shown	Sodium mg	Fat grams	Carbohy-drate grams	Calories
Salt—1 teaspoon				
Garlic or seasoned	1,850	.1	.7	4
Table, iodized	1,938	0	0	0
Sugar; granulated, 1 teaspoon	trace	0	4.0	16
Jam or preserves, 1 table-spoon	2	trace	14.0	54
Jelly, 1 tablespoon	3	trace	12.7	49
Sauces—1 tablespoon				
Barbecue sauce	130	1.7	1.2	15
Catsup	177	.1	4.3	19
Mustard, brown	352	1.7	1.4	25
Mustard, yellow	337	1.2	1.7	20
Soy sauce	1,209	.2	1.5	8
Tartar sauce	99	8.1	.6	74
Olives—canned, 2 large				
Green	61	1.0	.2	10
Black	38	.9	.1	9
Pickles				
Dill; 1 (4 x 1-3/4 inches)	1,924	.3	3.0	15
Sweet; 1 gherkin (1-1/2 ounces)	128	.2	18.0	73
Sweet relish (1 tablespoon)	107	trace	5.1	21

*Varies according to brand. Compiled from *The Dieter's Companion*,[66] *Nutrition Almanac*,[86] and *Tufts University Diet and Nutrition Letter* (December 1985).

Beverages to Be Sipped with Discretion

Alcoholic libations, coffee, tea, and caffeine-containing soft drinks have a mild diuretic action, so do little to replenish fluids lost through excretion and perspiration. Soft drinks contain sugar or artificial sweeteners of questionable virtue, plus phosphorus that can reduce the body's absorption of calcium unless quaffed in moderation.

ALCOHOL. For those who enjoy imbibing a bit of the bubbly, there are encouraging words:

- A six-year study involving 16,000 men (reported in the September 1989 issue of the *Atlantic*) revealed that those free of coronary heart disease consumed from 33 to 100 percent more alcohol than the men who were stricken.

- According to *Better Nutrition* (March 1987), supplements of vitamin C help prevent alcoholic liver cirrhosis.

- A study reported in *American Health* (July/August 1988) refutes earlier assumptions indicating an association between drinking and breast cancer.

However, besides the horrors of overindulgence, other alcoholic negatives remain. Its nonnutritious calories can be converted to energy by the liver but if not immediately used for that purpose are stored as fat and may raise cholesterol levels. Alcohol diminishes the body's B-vitamin supply, decreases the absorption of calcium, and, according to the *University of California, Berkeley Wellness Letter* (March 1989), stimulates the liver's production of harmful LDL cholesterol.

1 jigger (1-1/2 ounces) distilled liquor = 100 calories

1 can (12 ounces) regular beer = 150 calories

1 can (12 ounces) light beer = 70 to 120 calories

4 ounces champagne = 84 calories

4 ounces dry wine = 102 calories

4 ounces sweet wine = 165 calories

COFFEE AND CAFFEINE. Dr. Arthur Heller explains in *Shape* (September 1987) that it requires 75 cups of coffee to supply a lethal dose; but caffeine is present in many beverages besides coffee, is addictive, and is controversial. One to three cups of coffee a day can stimulate the nervous system, increase mental alertness, and lessen fatigue; and caffeine has been absolved of earlier charges associating it with birth defects, cancer, and fibrocystic breast lumps (*Health*, November 1987). Too much caffeine, however, constricts blood vessels, depletes calcium supplies, speeds up respiratory and heart action, causes irregular heartbeat, and instigates irritability, twitching muscles, and insomnia.

Decaffeinated Coffee: Removing the caffeine dispenses with most of coffee's suspected or acknowledged dangers, but both regular and decaf increase the secretion of stomach acid which can initiate indigestion or aggravate ulcers.

CAFFEINE CONTENT OF BEVERAGES*

per serving	Milligrams of caffeine
Coffee—6-ounce cup	
drip	130–180
perked	120–140
instant	70–100
Tea—6-ounce cup	
steeped 2 to 5 minutes	20–100
instant	40–60
Colas and caffeine-containing soft drinks, 12-ounce can	30–70
Hot cocoa, 6-ounce cup	5–35

*Varies with strength and brand. Compiled from *Earl Mindell's Shaping Up With Vitamins*,[108] *Eat Better, Live Better*[63] and *Managing Your Mind and Mood Through Food*.[183]

TEA. Steeping time regulates potency as well as flavor; shortening the brewing time to one minute can reduce the caffeine to ten milligrams per cup. Besides caffeine, pekoe contains tannin (an astringent that can irritate an empty stomach).

Herbal teas: These beverages should be imbibed judiciously. Foxglove is the equivalent of digitalis; Indian hemp is the original name for marijuana; ginseng is a more potent stimulant than caffeine; carcinogens have been detected in sassafras; the alkaloids in comfrey root have been linked to liver cancer; and cathartic herbs (aloe, buckthorn, dock root, senna leaves) can cause diarrhea.

Most herbal teas are beneficial. There are antioxidant herbs (rosemary is more effective than BHA and BHT); beautifying herbs (see Sections I and II); soothing, sleep-inducing herbs (camomile, catnip, dandelion, hops, lobelia, valerian); and energizing teas brewed from blackberry or raspberry leaves, cardamom, ginger, ginseng, goldenseal, lemon balm, rosemary, sage, or yerba mate.

How to Tailor Your Own "Look Beautiful, Feel Great" Diet

Nowhere is it graven in stone that we must eat three meals a day with specific foods at each one. Although *when* you consume *which* portion of your daily quota of nutrients doesn't affect their beautifying properties, it does affect your mental acuity and energy level. With either home-prepared or commercially produced natural foods you can tailor your own "look beautiful, feel great" diet to provide peak energy when you need it, keep your blood sugar and disposition on an even keel, and summon the sandman at day's end.

- **Protein foods** increase alertness by stimulating the brain's production of mentally energizing chemicals from the amino acid, tyrosine.
- **Complex carbohydrates** from fruits, vegetables and whole grains are the most efficient energy source.
- **Simple carbohydrates** from sugar and refined flours give a "quick fix" injection of energy, then trigger the "wearies" by releasing insulin and serotonin.
- **Fats** slow digestion, thus creating mental lethargy by diverting blood away from the brain to the stomach.
- **Excess calories** do more than produce bulges. Ingesting over 600 of them at one sitting lulls both body and soul—witness the living-room loungers after a family Thanksgiving dinner.

How to adapt your diet to your lifestyle

Cramming all your food-group servings into one meal a day would be impossible and unhealthful; eating several times during the day bolsters biological rhythms. Eating between meals is no longer frowned upon, and some health experts recommend a "grazing diet" consisting of nutritious snacks spaced throughout the day like an ongoing progressive meal.

The generally accepted pattern calls for eating approximately one fourth of the day's allotment within three hours of awakening. Unless a siesta is on your agenda, a high-protein 300-calorie lunch is advisable. For normal evenings, fill in any missing food-group servings or category percentages, and let your bathroom scale be your guide. If you need to remain dynamic for several more hours, dine on modest portions of high-protein, complex-carbohydrate foods and save the soporifics for a bedtime snack, or until you are ready to relax.

How to Supplement Your Diet
with Vitamins and Minerals

Food-group and category-percentage diets are designed to supply the recommended daily allowance (RDA) of vitamins and minerals. And they do—on paper. In reality, what you see on food- composition charts is not necessarily what your body gets. Soil depletion or production and preparation methods may leave one carrot without any vitamin A, its apparently identical twin with 5,000 IUs; some apricots are rich in A, iron, and copper; some aren't.

Dr. Walter Mertz, director of the U.S.D.A. Nutrition Research Center, explains in *American Health* (November 1985), that RDAs are based on the amounts required to prevent deficiency diseases, not on the levels needed to protect against stress, "environmental insults," and premature aging. Health scientists agree that a perfectly balanced, all-natural diet (organically grown vegetables, whole-grain breadstuffs) can fulfill these RDAs with as little as 1,200 calories a day. For a "reasonably sensible" diet, they estimate that 2,500 to 3,000 calories are needed; and admit that bodily assimilation of nutrients averages about 75 percent, even less when metabolic processes slow with increasing age.

Acquiring all the nutrients possible from natural dietary sources is important because man-made products are not always equivalent substitutes. We can't match Mother Nature's delicate balance of interacting elements (witness the enrichment of flour which replaces only 6 of the 22 nutrients removed during refining[109]).

Supplements provide insurance against deficiencies. Conservative physicians recommend a daily multivitamin-mineral tablet if you are on a restricted diet, pregnant or lactating, or are over 50; and many believe that the RDA for calcium may be too low to prevent bone loss (osteoporosis). Vitamin zealots claim fantastic benefits from megadoses that can be dangerous unless used as therapy under expert guidance. Although only fat-soluble vitamins A, D, E, and K are stored by the body, too much of anything, even if basically health-promoting, can disrupt nature's balance to create hypervitaminosis or deficiencies of interacting vitamins. Nutritionally oriented doctors and health specialists believe everyone should take a "multiple," plus individual supplements, at one or two meals each day. They also advise that, when embarking on a program of supplementation, the minimal amounts be taken at the beginning.

The external and internal benefits of specific vitamins and minerals, as well as their RDAs, are shown on the Vitamin and Mineral Chart, and the amounts suggested for enhancing beauty are given in Sections I and II. For optimum health and energy, daily supplements recommended are as follow:

A comprehensive multivitamin-mineral, preferably a two-a-day formula that divides the total RDAs for assimilation with morning and evening meals.

A = 25,000 IU in the form of beta carotene which the body transforms into vitamin A only when needed.

B = 1 or 2 stress tabs with the full complement of Bs.

C = 500 milligrams to 10,000 milligrams. Dr. Linus Pauling[122] extends the upper limit to 18 grams for combating colds or stress. Vitamin C is most effective when taken in divided doses containing or accompanied by bioflavonoids.

D = 400 IU to 4,000 IU. This "sunshine vitamin" is essential for assimilation of vitamin A and calcium, so the amount required depends on the amount of those two ingested. Fluid milk is fortified in the required ratio of 400 IU vitamin D to the 5,000 IU of vitamin A and approximately 1,200 milligrams of calcium in each quart.

E = 30 IU to 800 IU. Polyunsaturated oils contain vitamin E, yet require additional amounts to prevent its oxidation within the body. If you have diabetes, high blood pressure, or have ever had rheumatic fever, check with your physician before taking more than 100 IUs per day.

If your multivitamin-mineral supplement contains 18 milligrams of iron and 15 milligrams of zinc, plus other minerals, you may require only additional calcium. *The Secret of Youth*, a 1989 report published by The Lafayette Institute for Basic Research in Charlottesville, Virginia, advises reversing the accepted ratio of calcium and magnesium, and limiting daily calcium intake to 400 milligrams (plus 800 milligrams of magnesium) to prevent the calcification of soft body tissues which they believe results in premature aging. However, to forestall the osteoporosis which can shrink males as well as females, most experts advise a daily total of 1,200 milligrams of calcium—increased to 2,000 milligrams for postmenopausal women—balanced with no more than 1,000 milligrams of magnesium.

❧ 16 ❧

Beautiful Moves: How to Have Fun While You Exercise

Amid 1890's advertisements for constricting corsets and smelling salts to ward off fainting spells, ladies' magazines warned their gentle readers that perfect health could not be attained through enervating indolence. Now that the feminine ideal of languorous fragility has been replaced by one of radiant vitality, achieving a combination of beauty and health calls for more than external pampering and internal nourishing—it requires the movement of 696 muscles. The body keeps 200 of them in tone by cardiovascular and digestive functions; moving the rest is up to us. And not all the beautiful moves can be classed as "exercise."

Breathing Techniques That Beautify and Revitalize

To experience our full potential, most of us need more oxygen. With "normal" shallow breathing, only the upper portion of the lungs is utilized and less than a sixth of the air in our lungs is changed with each breath. Consciously controlled deep breathing promotes oxygenation of the blood and elimination of waste carbon monoxide. Just a few deep breaths each hour can have a beautifying, revitalizing effect. To evaluate your present lung capacity:

- Exhale and measure the circumference of your chest at the level of the breastbone. Inhale deeply and remeasure. Physical fitness expert Nicholas Kounovsky[89] says the expansion increase should be 2-1/2 inches for women, 3-1/2 inches for men.
- Watch a second hand while taking a deep breath and holding it as long as possible (55 seconds is average). Exhale and wait as long as you can before taking another breath (15 seconds is average).

Complete breathing requires slow inhalation of air into the lower lobes of the lungs by expanding the stomach area, then slow exhalation to expel stale air by tightening the diaphragm. Hatha yoga breathing calls for inhaling for a count of 8, holding your breath for a count of 4, then exhaling for a count of 8. A variation, called "healing breath," consists of breathing in for a count of 3, holding your breath for a count of 12, then breathing out for a count of 6. To strengthen your breathing muscles and acquire more oxygen:

- Whenever convenient, count as you breathe. Inhale normally and exhale twice as long as you inhaled.
- While walking, inhale for 3 or 4 steps and exhale for 6 or 8 steps. After a few weeks you can deepen your breathing by inhaling for 5 or 6 steps, exhaling for 10 or 12.

Looking Good: The Right Way to Stand Up

Actresses employ a stoop-shouldered, heat-thrust-forward, abdomen-protruding stance to portray elderly crones. "Standing tall" with head erect, back straight and stomach pulled in, reverses the effect. Besides being unattractive, poor posture is unhealthful for men as well as women. When shoulders hunch and the spine curls, the body's scrunched-up organs cannot function properly and waistlines thicken.

Uncomfortable rigidity, however, isn't necessary. Imagining yourself as a manikin manipulated by a puppeteer can ease the strain of maintaining young-looking posture. For effortless erectness, think string plus balloon. From the moment you arise, imagine that a helium-filled balloon is attached to the middle of your skull, supporting your weight. Let your arms and shoulders relax comfortably while your stomach flattens and your chin lifts. When walking with your weight-carrying balloon in place, swinging your legs from the hip joints rather than from the knees will present the smoothly elegant stride of native water-bearers or models who practice with books balanced on their heads.

How to Sit Tall

In our world of *homo sedentarius,* sitting is what we do most, but not necessarily best. It takes millenniums for evolutionary alterations to become operative, and chairs were introduced just 5,000 years ago as status symbols for kings and priests. So far, the only adaptation is derrier spread—each seat at the La Scala in Milan was recently widened 5 inches! Studies indicate that maximum comfort is achieved when body weight is shared between the feet and the hips, or when legs and feet are elevated.

- A back support and your imaginary helium-filled balloon can relieve the discomfort of "sitting up straight." Elevating your feet, or one foot at a time, on a 6-inch footstool concealed beneath your desk helps prevent the back strain that can result from hours of nonphysical labor.
- A chair with adjustable seat-height can be helpful. Hunching over a desk not only encourages the development of a double chin, it creates internal imbalances in the neck, back, and hips.
- Crossing your legs is neither injurious or varicose-vein producing if you restrict the crossing to ankle level or raise them to a "high crossing" (when suitably attired) of one ankle resting on the knee of the other leg.
- Pumping a rocking chair back and forth is excellent therapy for an aching back, ups blood circulation in your feet, and stimulates muscles in the lower leg.

How to Make Little Moves for Big Benefits

A balanced diet provides the wherewithal for beauty, health and energy, but our sedentary lifestyles create a vicious cycle; poor circulation which deprives skin, hair, and nails of needed nutrients; muscle deterioration; sluggish metabolism that piles on the pounds; and listless lethargy that overwhelms natural buoyancy. Muscle movement is an investment in energy that pays dividends of increased mental alertness and physical well-being, and offers a bonus benefit. It burns calories. The more calories we burn, the more nutritious food we can ingest without gaining weight; and the more vibrantly beautiful we become.

Internal metabolic processes require approximately 50 calories per hour while we are sleeping, sitting, or standing. Every little move increases caloric consumption and potential energy; avoiding movement can have the opposite effect. A systems analyst gained 6 pounds during the first six months following a promotion that entitled her to a garage parking space next to the elevator instead of one on the outskirts of the lot. She analyzed and remedied the problem by getting off the elevator two floors below her office and stair-climbing the rest of the way every morning and noon.

According to a report in *American Health* (May 1987), exercising enough to burn 2,000 calories a week improves fitness and extends life. To use up 100 calories you can swim one-third of a mile, walk one mile, bicycle four miles, or simply make the most of each daily activity. You don't have to participate in marathons or work out with sophisticated health-club equipment to be physically fit. Ordinary, everyday moves can be parlayed into an amazing amount of calorie-consumption; studies show that consistent, moderate exercise increases longevity more than rigorous athletic training.[94]

- Climbing stairs for 5 minutes burns 73 calories; descending stairs, 28.
- Typing on an electric typewriter or computer keyboard uses 105 calories per hour.
- "Light" housework uses 180 calories per hour; washing windows or scrubbing floors, 225. (As a result of extensive studies, Russian gerontologists arrived at an unsurprising conclusion: women live longer than men because they rarely retire from active work.[115])

Without counting either minutes or caloric expenditures, there are countless ways to extend your use of personal energy and keep your muscles supple.

- Use footpower instead of horsepower: get off the bus at the stop before your destination, walk up one or two flights of stairs instead of taking the elevator or escalator, park at the far end of the shopping mall rather than in front of the store.
- Use hand power instead of electric power: resurrect your potato masher and rotary egg beater, hand-chop the soup or salad vegetables, wash and dry those few dishes without waiting to fill the dishwasher.
- Move your legs while you stand and wait or work: wherever you are, rise up on your toes and rock down on your heels. At

the ironing board or kitchen sink, alternate side leg lifts and back kicks with marching in place.

- Make the most of every move: bend and stretch from the waist when making beds or retrieving small objects from the floor. Place frequently used supplies on high shelves so you stretch to reach them. Racewalk or jog from room to room. Bend one knee at a time and lunge like a fencer while vacuuming.

Three quick exercises you can do at home or in the office

Muscles tire from lack of movement as well as from exertion. Exercising for a few seconds relaxes and invigorates a chair- weary body:

- Stand tall, lift your arms above your head and lightly clasp your hands. With your head centered between your arms, bend to the right, swing across to the left, then return to the starting position. Repeat in the opposite direction.

- While standing, slowly lift one knee toward your chest; clasp both hands around the knee to pull it up and in as far as possible without strain. Deep breathe in and out. Release your hands and lower your knee. Repeat twice with each leg.

- Lean against a wall with your arms straight out in front, your back flat against the wall, and your heels as close to it as is comfortable. Lift your arms to touch the wall above your head, then swing them down to your sides as if making angels in the snow. Repeat three times.

Secret maneuvers: how to exercise while sitting

When standing isn't feasible, exercise while sitting down. If no one is watching, do a slow neck roll or extend both arms and flap your hands. If you have an audience, perform out-of-sight moves so that only your muscles will know and benefit.

- Rotate your ankles, then rock from heels to toes.

- Sit tall and tighten your stomach muscles. Place your palms on the desktop and slowly lift one leg at a time for a count of 5; relax for 5 seconds, then press both feet on the floor with as much force as possible for 5 seconds.

- Tense your left buttock for 5 seconds; relax for 5 seconds. Repeat with the right side, then tense both at the same time.

- Press your hands into your thighs for 5 seconds, relax for a count of 5; then pull up on your thighs for 5 seconds without raising your hands.

Stay-a-bed stretches

Shortly after the turn of the century, Sanford Bennett published *Exercise in Bed* (Hilton 1907) containing an hour-long series of movements to tone and rejuvenate the entire body. In October 1987, Tara Bennett-Goldman reported in *American Health* and *Good Housekeeping* that in-bed exercises help readjust the circulatory system and muscles from horizontal relaxation to vertical activity. Moving like a sleek cat for three reps of each exercise in the following three-minute morning motivator can get you going before you get out of bed. Just throw back the covers, lie flat on your back, and begin.

1. Slowly stretch your arms above your head, your toes to the foot of the bed.
2. Stretch both arms toward the ceiling, spread your fingers, tense and curl them like a cat's claws; then fling your arms out and bring them back so your palms press together.
3. Clasp your hands behind your head and bend your knees to place your feet flat, 10 inches apart. Pull your pubic bone toward your navel while pressing with your feet and raising your hips. Slowly lower your hips and straighten your knees.
4. Raise your right knee to your chest, clasp it with both hands and pull it toward your chin. Slowly lower your knee against the pressure of your hands. Repeat with the left leg. Then draw both knees to your chest and hold them with your arms. Tense your stomach muscles and gently rock your knees from side to side.
5. Bend your left knee to place the heel on your right thigh. Grasp your left ankle with your right hand and gently pull the heel up your thigh until moderate tension develops. Hold for 20 seconds. Repeat with the opposite leg.

The Six-minute Shape-up Guide
for Toning and Limbering

A lithe body with firm, resilient muscles is our prerogative regardless of age. There is no biological reason for body fat to increase while muscle and bone tissue decrease at the current rate of 1 percent each two years. Hippocrates' observation, "That which is used develops, that which is not used wastes away," is particularly applicable to joints and muscles. If not exercised, joints stiffen, muscles weaken, and flab develops. As little as six minutes a day of proper exercise can reverse this process, shape up the body, and restore youthful bounce and glow. The "shaping up" is automatic. A pound of fat occupies 20 percent more space than a pound of muscle, yet requires fewer calories for maintenance. By exercising, you can exchange bulges for sleek sinew and wear a smaller size without losing any weight. If you are dieting to lose pounds, exercise not only speeds fat loss by burning extra calories, it also prevents muscle loss and saggy skin.

How to move safely

Recent fitness enthusiasm has led to reevaluation of the therapeutic benefits and the possible pitfalls of exercise. New-and-improved exercises have been developed to replace strenuous calisthenics that can be hazardous to joints and muscles.

- **Deep-knee bends and duck walking** are no longer recommended because they put too much strain on the knees.
- **Bent-knee hang downs,** performed slowly, without force or jerky bouncing (which can cause microscopic tears in muscles) replace the locked-knee toe touches that overstress back, knees, and hamstring muscles.
- **Bent-leg raise-ups,** with the lower back pressed into the floor, arms crossed over the chest or behind the head and shoulders raised only high enough to clear the floor, replace straight-leg sit-ups that place excessive stress on the lower back and hip flexor muscles.
- **Single leg lifts,** with one knee bent and foot flat on the floor, are safer than double leg lifts that overstress the lower back.
- **Rear thigh lifts,** while on all fours, with the thigh slowly brought up parallel to the torso and the knee bent to form a right angle, safely work buttock muscles without the back strain or neck and shoulder contortions of the old "donkey kicks," which called for rapidly lifting one leg as high as possible.

Before embarking on any exercise program it is wise to have a medical checkup. If your arteries have hardened you may need to exercise in a horizontal position because blood vessels expand naturally when you are on a level plane; when you exercise in a standing position, your heart must pump blood uphill through forcibly expanded blood vessels over 70 times every minute.[112]

- *Start slowly.* Begin your regimen by performing each exercise only twice, then gradually work up to the desired total. Starting each session with slow moves allows your muscles to warm up. A warm shower increases muscle flexibility by as much as 20 percent. Exercising in front of an air conditioner or in 65- degree air can reduce the range of motion by 10 to 20 percent.

- *Let your digestive organs do their job* before drawing their needed blood away to move other muscles. Twenty minutes is considered essential to avoid possible indigestion or cramping, an hour is better. Exercising before a meal is ideal because it may decrease your appetite and improve your digestion.

- *Use an exercise mat or a carpeted surface* for all seated or prone-position exercises. (Beds do not offer sufficient support for exercises other than the stay-a-bed stretches.)

- *Breathe while you move.* Inhale with the easy move; exhale with the difficult one; holding your breath strains the cardiovascular system.

- *Move at your own pace.* Professionals may move faster than you should; slow and sinuous movement is best for improving flexibility, smooth and rhythmic for muscle toning.

- *Individualize your full-body program* by selecting several exercises from both of the following categories. Build up to the number of repetitions needed to reach your goal: 6 reps of each for a total of 6 minutes a day to maintain flexibility and muscle tone; 10 reps of each for a total of 12 minutes to stretch and strengthen muscles.

  If you have a sturdy door with a firmly anchored doorknob, you can add this allover conditioner: grasp one side of the knob with each hand, keep your tummy tucked in, your back and arms straight while you slowly squat until your hips touch your heels, then slowly pull yourself up to a standing position.

- *Exercise with a partner* to add the pleasure of companionship and to maintain a consistent regimen. Melanie and Carl are a case in point. Although she hadn't gained weight, time and gravity were increasing the circumference of Melanie's waist. She had been exercising sporadically, but her busy schedule and waning enthusiasm always provided excellent excuses for putting her after-work firming-up program on hold. When she dissolved in tears because Carl had to help zip her into the sung-fitting dress that had "shrunk" while hanging in the closet, he came up with the solution. "Let's set the alarm fifteen minutes earlier in the morning and shape up together. My belts are getting a little tight, too." Clothes now fit the way they should, and neither Carl nor Melanie is tempted to forsake their slightly competitive few minutes of before-breakfast camaraderie.

Upper body exercises

- Stand with your feet wide apart. Fold your arms in front of your waist and cup each elbow with the hand of the other arm. Slowly raise your folded arms over your head as far back as possible without discomfort, then slowly lower them to the starting position.

- Stand with your arms straight out in front, palms down. Bend your elbows down to raise your hands, palms up, directly above your shoulders. Slowly raise both palms straight up as though you were lifting a heavy box. Hold the imaginary box steady for a few seconds before slowly lowering it and returning to the starting position.

- Stand with hands loosely clasped behind your back. Keep your arms straight while slowly bringing your elbows as close together as possible without strain.

- Lie face down with your knees bent, ankles crossed, and your feet raised several inches. Bend your elbows and place your palms flat on the floor under your shoulders, fingers pointed inward. Keep your head and torso in a straight line while slowly pushing up until your arms are fully extended to share the weight with your knees. Slowly lower your body almost to the floor and push back up again.

Middle and lower body exercises

For maximum benefit, complete the repetitions for each separate exercise before going on to the next one in a group of complementary exercises such as this first one.

- Stand tall with feet 24 inches apart, arms outstretched at shoulder level. Twist at the waist to reach forward, then backward with each arm.

  Lower your left arm and slide it down to your knee as you bend to the left and raise your right arm. Reverse to bend to the right.

Leave your feet in position, bend forward from the waist (without locking knees) and let your arms swing loosely between your legs for 10 seconds—with fingers curled if your hands touch the floor.

- Sit with knees bent, feet flat on the floor, and arms folded in front of your chest. Keep your spine straight while you lean back until you feel the abdominal muscles tighten. Hold for 5 seconds before returning to the starting position.

Straighten your arms and place your hands flat on the floor behind you. Straighten and raise your right leg, then bend the right knee and slip the right foot under your left knee without touching the floor. Straighten the right leg, return to the starting position. Relax and repeat with the opposite legs.

- Lie on your back with hands under your head. With knees bent, toes pointed, and both feet clear of the floor, raise your head and alternate legs while twisting to touch the right knee with the left elbow, left knee with right elbow.

- Lie on your back with knees up, feet flat on the floor, and arms crossed over your chest with the fingertips at shoulder level. Press down with your lower back while slowly raising your head and shoulders toward your knees until your shoulder blades are clear of the floor, then lower to the starting position.

As an alternative: Lie on the floor with your hips close to the legs of a straight chair, your feet and calves resting on the chair seat. Grasp the bottom of the chair legs with your hands and slowly pull yourself up until your shoulders are raised. Keep your lower back in contact with the floor while returning to the starting position.

- Lie on your back with knees bent, arms at your sides, palms down. Slowly raise your legs and pelvis off the floor until your knees are almost over your fact. Return to the starting position.

Leave your hands at your sides. Lift and straighten your legs over your hips. Slowly separate your legs as wide as possible without strain, then bring them back together.

- With knees slightly flexed, bend over and place your palms on the floor. Without raising your head, walk on all fours as if you were a primordial creature.

Drop to your knees, leave your arms extended, and round your back up for a count of 5. Rock back so your hips are over your heels, slide your arms out in front of you, and rest your forehead on the floor for 5 seconds.

Heartfelt Moves: 11 Benefits of Aerobic Exercise

Stop-and-go sports and exercises such as those in the preceding sections improve flexibility and help you keep trim. EMS (Electronic Muscle Stimulators) help rehabilitate muscles damaged by severe accident or disease but, as explained in the February 1989 issue of *Mayo Clinic Nutrition Letter*, they will not make you either beautiful or fit. A regular program of continuously sustained aerobic activities (walking, swimming, rowing, etc.) maintain vibrant beauty and health by strengthening the cardiovascular system and deepening breathing to provide more oxygen, and offer an extensive array of potential rewards.

1. **Alleviated tension and elevated mood.** Sustained movement at target heart rate causes your body to produce greater amounts of the beta-endorphins which counter stress and depression, increase tolerance to pain, and account for the euphoric "runner's high."

2. **Aroused alertness.** A 30-minute bout of aerobic exercise has been shown to improve short-term memory and increase mental performance by 25 percent.[93]

3. **Better regulated blood-sugar levels.** Physical activity improves glucose tolerance and reduces insulin resistance. If you have diabetes, however, be sure to check with your doctor before beginning an aerobic regimen; it might trigger hemorrhaging if you suffer from retinopathy.

4. **Extended lifespan.** A 17,000-person study being conducted by Stanford Medical School indicates that each hour of aerobic activity increases anticipated longevity; by 1.95 hours if you are 40 years old; by 2.61 hours if you are 60.

5. **Improved skin tone.** Regular exercise slows cell degeneration and collagen breakdown (the prime instigators of wrinkling) and keeps your skin glowingly healthy because of the extra oxygen and nutrients provided through stimulated blood circulation.

6. **Increased energy.** As explained in *Mayo Clinic Nutrition Newsletter* (October 1988), energy levels increase as the body adapts to exercise, muscles become better able to utilize oxygen, the heart's pumping capacity improves, and the resting pulse slows. The average resting heart rate is 78 per minute, with a variance of 10 considered normal. By conditioning your heart through exercise, you can reduce the resting rate to 70 or less, which allows your heart to pump the same amount of blood with fewer beats.

7. **Lowered blood pressure and cholesterol.** Habitual aerobic exercise has been shown to bring about a dramatic drop in hypertension and elevated cholesterol levels, along with an increase of the blood substance that dissolves heart-attack- instigating clots.[32, 115] A report in the March 1988 issue of American Health states that the proportion of "good" HDL cholesterol is raised when you walk or run 12 miles each week at any pace; achieving your target heart rate is not essential to this benefit.

8. **Reduced weight and girth.** In addition to immediately decreasing appetite, eight to twelve minutes of aerobic activity contributes to weight loss by burning between 80 and 200 calories, boosts the metabolic rate so that you continue to burn calories at a higher rate for up to two days, and builds lean tissue which occupies less space than the replaced fat, thus reducing your inches.

9. **Relieved PMS.** Regular exercise has an effect on female hormones that may prevent or abate premenstrual tension and water retention.

10. **Stimulated immune system.** According to worldwide tests reported in Prevention (February 1988), the amount of virus- and cancer-fighting lymphocytes in the blood are more than doubled by an hour of bicycle riding or other moderate aerobic activity. Overly intensive training, however, can hamper immunity; with the exception of daily walks, you should adhere to the classic recommendation of three to four 30-minute aerobic sessions per week.

11. **Stronger bones.** Studies conducted at the University of Oregon indicate that a program of regular exercise increases bone density to offset the decline in bone mass which normally commences after the age of 40. Developing peak bone mass through exercise and adequate calcium consumption before the age of 35 protects against osteoporosis later in life; consistent postmenopausal exercise plus calcium can replace lost bone density.

How to target your heart rate

The heart's ability to speed up with exercise diminishes so predictably that "maximum heart rate" has been established as 220 minus a person's age. Numerous studies show that the "normal" decline in cardiac capacity can be combated by any activity that brings the heart rate into the target zone of 60 to 80 percent of its maximum and maintains it from 5 to 20 minutes. The least complex method of targeting your heart-rate goal is to subtract your age from 220, then multiply that total by the desired percentage. For instance: if you are 40 years old, your target heart rate would be 126 (220 minus 40 = 180 multiplied by .70); the acceptable "low" would be 108, the "high," 144.

If you don't have an electronic pulse monitor, you can check your heart rate by pausing while exercising, placing your left middle fingers next to your windpipe or over the pulse on your right wrist, counting it for 6 seconds, then multiplying by 10. (The medical practice of counting for 15 seconds and multiplying by 4 is impractical during exercise because the heartbeat slows rapidly when physical activity is discontinued.)

Eight Ways to Avoid Aerobic Adversities

Before embarking on any fitness program, it is wise to obtain your physician's approval, then:

1. *Schedule your aerobic sessions several hours after eating so your digestive system is not disrupted.* "Carbohydrate loading" an hour before exercising is no longer advocated even for competitive athletes.[93]

2. *Warm up first.* When your body is at rest, approximately 85 percent of your blood supply is in your chest and abdomen. As activity begins, blood moves to the working muscles which then "heat up" to such an extent that they could boil a quart of water in an hour. If your muscles are abruptly required to stretch and squeeze to their limit, ligaments may tighten around joints and, in extreme cases, muscles can tear. Studies reveal that 60 percent of sports injuries are traceable to improper warm-up techniques.[70]

The length of your warm-up and the movements involved depend on your starting condition and the type of exercise. If you have been up and moving, going for a walk will entail no warm-up. If you plan to leap out of bed and onto your bike for a 15-minute spin, play fair with your muscles by performing some limbering exercises. Then begin your aerobic activity at low intensity; walk before you run, swim a slow lap instead of diving in and breast-stroking at top speed.

3. *Cool down.* Allowing your muscles a cooling off period is as crucial as warming them up. Abruptly stopping a workout can cause a sudden drop in blood pressure that may produce dizziness plus blood pooling and an aftermath of painfully tight muscles. Gradually slowing your activity for the final 5 minutes (or performing mild stretching and bending exercises after a bout of rope jumping or other activity that does not lend itself to low intensity) permits a return to normalcy without danger.

If you have been perspiring heavily, wait for your temperature to drop before showering. A cool shower will shock your system; a hot one can draw so much blood to the skin that there might not be enough left to supply your internal organs. If you've overexercised, a tub-bath herbal soak of juniper or lemon balm often relieves the worst of the muscle pain.

4. *Approach your aerobic goals sensibly.* Consistency is the key to muscle conditioning; strengthening occurs during the 48 hours following vigorous exercise. If the activity is not repeated within 72 hours, muscles begin to shrink and lose their new-found flexibility at the rate of about 1 percent per day.

The standard regimen calls for three or four weekly sessions of approximately 30 minutes each (5 to 10 minutes for warm up, 12 to 20 minutes at target heart rate, 5 to 10 minutes to cool down). Research reported in *University of California, Berkeley Wellness Letter* (November 1988) indicates that "interval training" of 3 to 5 minutes at target heart rate, 3 minutes of slowed-down activity (60-percent heart rate), then another 3 to 5 minutes at high intensity produces 10 percent greater gains in aerobic capacity than steady-speed sessions. Lower intensity, longer-duration activity forces the body to break down stored fat for energy.

5. *Put your program on hold if you have a fever or virus.* Elevating your temperature even higher by exercising can aggravate your illness, and viruses make muscle fibers more susceptible to tears and injuries.

6. *"Think" yourself into a successful regimen.* By remembering that you are working with Mother Nature to help your body—not striving to punish it or yourself—you can turn what might be a disagreeably boring workout into a pleasurable experience. Experiment until you discover which of these options works best for you: Mentally envision the eventual results of your efforts. Concentrate on your muscular movements while visualizing your body reshaping itself into more glamorous contours. Or, evolve a meditation-type mantra such as whispering "down" every time one foot hits the ground. Or, imagine an applauding audience admiring the grace and aplomb with which you whip through your exercise session. Or, disassociate yourself from the entire process by wearing a radio or tape-playing headset if outdoors, or by watching television while pedaling, rowing, skiing, or walking with indoor exercise equipment.

7. *Dress in comfortable clothing with properly fitted shoes designed for your chosen activity.* For outdoor activities in cold weather, wear gloves and a hat to hold heat in your body. In the summer, a white or light-colored hat will reflect the sun's rays. Leg warmers help avoid cramping by keeping your muscles warm, but rubber or plastic "condi-

tioning suits" can cause dehydration and deprive your skin of oxygen. (The pounds of liquid lost reappear as soon as you drink a few glasses of water; the harm to your system lingers.)

8. *Replenish fluids and nutrients.* Thirst is not always a reliable guide to Mother Nature's needs. Fluid losses from perspiration during strenuous activity can deplete your water-soluble vitamins and minerals as well as liquids. Sports medicine specialists advise drinking a glass of cool water 20 minutes before, at 20-minute intervals during, and immediately after exercising.[68] Nutritionists suggest a daily multivitamin-mineral supplement as insurance, extra vitamin E to protect cell membranes from destruction by oxidation from the increased oxygen intake,[164] and a diet rich in potassium-containing foods (see the Vitamin and Mineral Chart) to prevent leg cramps. Taking a 500-milligram vitamin-C-plus-bioflavonoids tablet before and after exercising is a muscle-stiffness preventive.

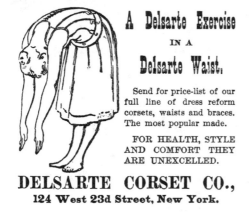

A Delsarte Exercise

IN A

Delsarte Waist,

Send for price-list of our full line of dress reform corsets, waists and braces. The most popular made.

FOR HEALTH, STYLE AND COMFORT THEY ARE UNEXCELLED.

DELSARTE CORSET CO.,
124 West 23d Street, New York.

Clothing should be even less confining than this whaleboned waist advertised in 1892.

Nine Aerobic Exercises That Strengthen the Cardiovascular System

Customizing your beautifying, cardiovascular-improving program can be as simple as getting up earlier and walking to work. If you prefer to move in the company of others, sign up for a class, join a club, or exercise with a friend. You can opt for a single activity or, with your muscles kept in shape by daily toning exercises, vary your program to avoid monotony. Aerobic dancing, cross-country skiing, cycling, jogging or running, rope jumping, rowing, swimming, walking—whatever works for you is "right" for your body as long as your doctor approves and you always warm up and cool down.

1. Aerobic dancing

Whether you participate in a class or work out in privacy with a video tape, aerobic dancing is a fun way to keep fit. Low Impact Aerobics (LIA or soft aerobics) have replaced the ballistic, bouncy routines that resulted in high injury rates. Wearing aerobic shoes with rearfoot and lateral support further lessens the possibility of shin splints or foot problems.

Calories burned: 60 to 90 each 10 minutes, depending on the intensity of activity.

2. Cross-country skiing

The movements required for cross-country skiing utilize muscles in the arms, legs, and trunk in equal measure, and are virtually free of injury-initiating stresses. Easily stored "ski machines" allow you to benefit from this aerobic exercise in the comfort of your own home, without waiting for the snow to fall.

Calories burned: 70 to 200 each 10 minutes, depending on tempo.

3. Cycling

Enthusiasm for this activity began in 1891 when the "safety bicycle" replaced prior models with their huge, unmanageable front wheels. If you live in an area where outdoor biking is feasible, our twentieth-century models offer designs for city, mountain, or all-terrain cycling. To alternate outdoor riding with indoor pedaling, you can put your bike up on rollers in your living room. If back-to-nature biking is impractical or undesirable (half an hour amid city traffic fills your lungs with as much carbon monoxide as ten cigarettes[128]), invest in a stationary exercycle which offers similar cardiovascular, upper-leg, and buttock-toning benefits.

Calories burned: 65 for each 10 minutes of pedaling at 10 mph with a heart rate of 130.

4. Jogging and running

Jogging is usually classified as running when the speed exceeds six miles an hour. Either activity is great for your heart, and for weight reduction, but both are so joint-jarring and injury-ridden they should be undertaken only with medical approval. Begin your program by alternating five minutes of brisk walking with five minutes of slow jogging, then gradually increase the jogging segments. Jog or run for your set period of time, not for distance or speed. The ideal pace is one that keeps your heart rate within the target zone while leaving you with enough breath to carry on a conversation. According to Dr. Thomas McMahon (*Prevention*, December 1987), bending your knees just ten extra degrees and taking "scurrying" steps emphasizes the role of thigh and buttock muscles, reduces the amount of shock transmitted through the body by 80 percent, and uses up 25 percent more calories than the customary gait.

Calories burned: 80 for 10 minutes of jogging at 5 miles per hour; 130 when running at 10 miles per hour.

5. Jumping rope

If you want to improve your cardiovascular system with the least expenditure of time, and you have your physician's approval, this is the ideal aerobic activity. The President's Council on Physical Fitness and Sports found five minutes of rope jumping the equal of fifteen minutes of jogging. Although it seems too good to be true, utilizing your six minutes of daily exercise as a warm-up; jumping for five minutes, five times a week; then doing walk-around household chores for two minutes while you cool down can take care of your fitness regimen.

Both *Joy of Jumping*[30] and *The Hop, Skip and Jump Way to Health*[110] recommend building up to 500 continuous jumps by beginning with 10 jumps per session several times a day. To ease into the program, jump one foot at a time; to increase the benefits, jump with both feet and jump higher than the suggested one inch off the floor. If your ceiling is too low, or if you don't have a rope, you can simulate by assuming the position (upper arms near the ribs, forearms at a 45 degree angle) and rotating your wrists while jumping.

Calories burned: 63 for each 5 minutes at 120 to 140 turns per minute.

6. Rowing

Whether stroking across the water in a shell or rowing a machine while watching television, this is a superb, full-body exercise. The popularity of home exercise equipment has led to multi-action combinations such as rower-cycles and rower-skiers that cost no more than membership in a fitness club. Rowing is an effective back-strengthener often prescribed for those with lower back and disk problems, but it is not suitable for certain physical conditions. Check with your doctor before experimenting.

Calories burned: 60 to 325 each 10 minutes, depending on intensity of activity.

7. Swimming

The buoyancy of water so reduces stress on joints and ligaments that swimming is a perfect exercise for the elderly or for anyone with physical problems, yet its muscle toning and aerobic benefits equal those of land-based activities. Body beautifying as well as cardiovascular-conditioning, swimming also bolsters bones. In *Clinical Research* (January 1987), Dr. Eric Orwoll cites tests showing that swimming is as efficient as weight-bearing exercise in building bone mass to retard osteoporosis.

Maximum heart rate for swimming is slower than for other activities because water absorbs body heat and the horizontal position eases blood circulation. To compute your 12-to 20-minute target zone: subtract your age from 205, then multiply by the desired percentage between 60 and 80. (For our 40-year-old, 125-pound example, this would be 115 at 70 percent of maximum heart rate.)

Calories burned: 50 to 115 each 10 minutes, depending on the vigor of exertion.

8. Walking

Although it may not seem like exercise, walking provides the same benefits as other aerobic activities, and can be practical as well as healthily beautifying. You can substitute your walks for riding (as in walking to work) or combine them with necessary errands. Carrying heavy objects or wearing ankle weights is not advisable because of the possibility of straining the body's joints by upsetting nature's balance between arms and legs; but hand weights of one to three pounds, designed for walkers or joggers, can safely be used to increase the effort.

Begin by "strolling" on alternate days, gradually increase your pace to raise your heart rate into its target zone for at least 12 minutes with a cadence of 90 to 120 steps per minute. For precise monitoring (and for fascinating diversion), splurge on a wristwatch-pulse counter and a pedometer. To avoid becoming overheated as your muscles warm up, dress for a temperature 10 to 20 degrees warmer than it actually is, then walk *with* the wind as you start out; *against* it as you return. Walking in a light drizzle or amid drifting snowflakes is delightful, but, if the weather outside is frightful or if your neighborhood is rife with potential danger from mortals or motor fumes, walk in the comfortable safety of a shopping mall or purchase a treadmill.

- *Strolling* (1–2 mph): burns approximately 30 calories each 10 minutes, seldom achieves target heart rate but lowers cholesterol and may be utilized as warm up and cool down for fitness walking.

- *Brisk walking* (3–3-1/2 mph, 50 calories per 10 minutes)

- *Striding* (3-1/2–5-1/2 mph, 50–75 calories per 10 minutes): long, swift strides expend almost as much energy as jogging, without the sometimes-injurious jarring impact.

- *Racewalking* (4–6 mph, 65–120 calories per 10 minutes): This full-body exercise uses the same number of muscles as swimming, and has become so popular with celebrities that its exaggerated hip-swing is regarded as sexy. Racewalking requires a warm-up and cool down of limbering exercises, plus mastery of its unique moves.

  1. Keep your feet close to the ground, reaching forward with one heel while pushing off with the toe of the other foot. Straighten the knee of the advancing leg as the pushing-off toe maintains ground contact until the reaching heel touches down so there is a split-second of double support.

  2. Rotate your pelvis to direct your movement in a straight line so your feet land directly in front of one another.

  3. Keep your hands in loose fists, your arms bent at right angles, and swing your elbows high—left arm and right leg forward, right arm and left leg back. Your shoulders should lift and lower with each stride; your head glide smoothly, parallel with the ground.

9. Oriental moves

For over six thousand years, Ch'i Kung, Dao Yin, T'ai Chi Ch'uan, Yeng Shu, Yoga and similar disciplines have been practiced by Far Eastern peoples. All adhere to the Taoist principle of mind-body unification and control to prevent and correct ailments, improve bodily functions, and reverse the aging process. The physical portions of two of these disciplines, T'ai Chi Ch'uan and Hatha Yoga, have been adopted by the Western world. Yoga is not sufficiently vigorous to accelerate the pulse into its target heart-rate zone, but both are excellent fitness exercises that benefit the cardiovascular system.

T'AI CHI CH'UAN: Originating in Tibet and perfected in China during the Sung Dynasty (960–1278 A.D.), T'ai Chi Ch'uan is now practiced daily by millions of Orientals who perform the 128 stylized, dancelike postures each dawn and dusk in a twenty-minute ritual of constant motion designed to allow the free flow of energies throughout the body. Usually referred to as T'ai Chi, it can be learned from illustrated texts such as *Knocking at the Gate of Life*[33] and *The Chinese Way to a Long and Healthy Life*[125] or by attending classes at health clubs, Y.M.C.A.s, and community centers. Condensed versions of T'ai Chi include fewer postures; at Rancho La Peurta in Mexico, the slow, smooth motions are completed in ten minutes to the accompaniment of Latin music.

The broad range of curative powers claimed by its adherents may be questioned by skeptics, but, although performed with deliberation, target heart rate can be achieved after only one minute of the exercise.[55] Pennsylvania's Swathmore College has incorporated T'ai Chi into its football team's training schedule, and an international lecturer testifies to its fitness and stamina building. On a tour of the Orient this 70-year-old became so intrigued by the early-morning sight of young and old Chinese performing T'ai Chi that she studied and regularly practiced the movements. The following year, she impressed herself and the men she hired to cut down one of her trees. For four hours, while they sawed the tree into logs for her fireplace, she picked up the wood, trundled it 30 yards in a wheelbarrow, unloaded and stacked it—and suffered no painful after-effects the next day.

HATHA YOGA: Even more ancient that T'ai Chi Ch'uan, Yoga has two distinct aspects. The spiritual side, concerned with knowledge and meditation, must be pursued under the guidance of a guru. The physical, Hatha Yoga, which emphasizes deep breathing and sinuous poses to foster flexibility and extend life, has achieved international acclaim. After the *asanas* (poses) have been mastered under the tutelage of an instructor, it can be practiced at home. (Because Hatha Yoga affects every part of the body, it is wise to check with your physician before attempting any of the advanced poses.)

In India, where it is regarded as a cure for everything from gout and wrinkles to sexual impotence and the common cold, each of the 25 Yoga centers in Delhi has a daily attendance of 1,500. In America, where Hatha Yoga classes are taught in health clubs, Y's, and senior centers, it is credited with almost as many bodily benefits; including increased stamina, relieved stress and tension, reduced bronchial difficulty, and improved musculature to alleviate lower back pain.[94]

❧ 17 ❧

Making the Least of Stress

Stress is Beauty Enemy Number 1. External appearance mirrors internal health—emotional as well as physical—and reflects stress reactions. Linked to the brain by thousands of nerve endings, skin not only blushes when we are embarrassed and pales when we are frightened, it can react to too much stress by drying out and itching or wrinkling; becoming too oily and erupting with blemishes; or by developing eczema, hives, or psoriasis.

How Stress and Illness Interact

The physical connection

In the 1960s, Doctors Holmes and Rahe devised a "Stressful Events Rating Chart" as an indicator of illness potential. On a scale of 1 to 100, the chart depicts receiving a traffic ticket (11 points) at the bottom; getting married, buying a house, being fired, or retiring (approximately 50 points each) in the middle; divorce (73 points) or the death of a spouse (100 points) at the top. If your total score for a 12-month period falls between 150 and 300, your chance of suffering serious illness is 53 percent; if your points exceed 300, the probability is 80 percent.

Further studies reveal that an accumulation of minor stresses can be equally hazardous—responsible for a myriad of apparently unrelated disorders such as arthritis, chronic fatigue, colitis, dandruff, dental caries, depression, hair loss, headaches, high blood pressure, indigestion, peeling fingernails, sexual dysfunction, tinnitus, and ulcers. Evolution's pokiness is at the root of these stress-induced misfortunes. Our bodies have not yet developed the ability to discriminate between a traffic snarl and the growl of a saber-tooth tiger entering the cave; they still react to stress with the "fight-or-flight" response.

1. Stress hormones—adrenaline, noradrenaline (epenephrine, norepinephrine), cortisol—are released to prepare the body for action.

2. Breathing becomes shallow and rapid; heartbeat, blood sugar, and cholesterol levels rise; digestive processes slow and practically come to a halt.

3. If the stress continues, or is not released after a brief period, the body resumes its most vital functions but remains on "red alert" (free-floating anxiety).

4. If unrelieved stresses occur frequently, the body becomes exhausted: accident prone, mentally inefficient and depressed, physically vulnerable to illness, and aesthetically unattractive.

The mental connection

Stress has almost as many definitions as it does causes and effects. In the health sciences, stress is defined as something that is (or is believed to be) a threat to the continuance of existing lifestyle. Any change, positive or negative, can trigger the stress response. Frustration is stress that comes when things don't turn out the way we want them to, when we feel thwarted, or when we lose control of our lives. (Studies reported in the August 1988 issue of *University of California, Berkeley Wellness Letter* reveal that lower echelon workers are more prone to stress-related problems than upper echelon decision makers.)

Our safe, civilized society abounds with stressors: long lines at check-out counters, ringing telephones and busy signals, computer glitches, the constant pressures of multi-faceted career and homemaker roles... Mental reaction to stress is a matter of individual perception. A stepped-up deadline may be a creative challenge to one person, a traumatic catastrophe to a co-worker. By identifying personal stress-triggers, avoiding or modifying as many as possible, and learning to demobilize physical reactions to stresses that cannot be altered, we can maintain an inner serenity that preserves our health and radiates vibrant beauty.

The nutritional connection

Diet, the third member of the stress-management triad, augments relaxation and exercise. Poor nutrition is in itself a stress, low blood sugar initiates the stress response, and physical or mental stress depletes essential nutrients—another vicious cycle in the making. By providing your body with a well-balanced diet (see Chapter 15) you can protect yourself against many of the harmful effects of stress, and the fatigue of its aftermath. Nutritionists and holistic physicians advise taking extra vitamin C (up to 1,000 milligrams per hour during extreme stress), and one to three B-complex tablets each day.

NATURAL TRANQUILIZERS: "Eat something; you'll feel better," is a folk-remedy truism with a factual nucleus. A bite or two of anything temporarily alleviates stress by providing a few moments of pleasurable self-gratification. Chewing or sipping substances that offset stress can give longer-lasting relief.

- Eating an ounce of gumdrops, jelly beans, or dry cereal without milk, can foil the fluttering butterflies in your midsection. Sweet, starchy carbohydrates (without fat, fiber, or protein to slow their assimilation) immediately prompt the body to secrete opiate-like endorphins as well as the serotonin that eases anxiety and tension. Ration them carefully—doubling the amount might put you to sleep.

- Drinking a cup of any of the herbal teas listed for encouraging sleep will help calm daytime nervousness. Herbalists suggest brewing up a mixture of equal parts of balm leaves, hops, lavender flowers, and primrose; and as reported in *Prevention* (September 1988), tests at Rutgers University show valerian to be an efficient tranquilizer with no side effects.

- Sipping half a cup of this "super milk" every few hours will calm your nerves, keep your blood sugar on an even keel, and help replenish the protein and potassium used up by stress reactions. Combine in an electric blender and whir until smooth:

  2 cups fluid lowfat milk

  1/2 cup instant nonfat dry milk

  1 sliced banana

  1 tablespoon brewer's yeast

Optional additions for increased benefits: 1 tablespoon lecithin granules, miller's bran, peanut butter, protein powder, *or* wheat germ.

- Taking dolomite or other calcium-magnesium tablets provides quick-acting, between-meals nerve-soothing. Tryptophan is another pill that can be popped with impunity; 500 milligrams taken an hour before or after meals has been found as effective as tranquilizing drugs.[108]

Six Ways to Dodge or Diminish Stressful Situations

An astounding amount of stress is self-instigated, or self-perpetuated, and, therefore, subject to self-destruction.

- Re-evaluating goals and establishing priorities often relieves the stress of trying too hard to achieve or acquire more than is needed or really wanted—and makes it easier to say "no." Saying "yes" to the best of friends or the worthiest of causes is foolish and stressful when it deprives you of high-priority family or private time.

- Guilt trips can be canceled when you accept the fact that no one is expected to be 100 percent perfect 100 percent of the time; make appropriate amends or apologies; and regard each gaffe or goof-up as a learning experience.

- Anger, disappointment, and frustration are seldom self-made, but their damaging effects can be limited by following the advice of ancient philosophers and modern psychologists: keep your head, perspective, and sense of humor; move on to something positive; and dissipate physical reactions through relaxation and exercise. Losing your "cool," devoting sleepless nights to ruminating over what you "shudda said," plotting revenge, or wallowing in your woes merely creates more stress.

- Worry can be either a stressor or a stress reliever. Utilizing "worrying time" to formulate a series of "just in case" alternatives eliminates debilitating "stewing" and leaves you confidently in control. If the disaster should occur, you are prepared; if plans A fails, you have plans B and C to fall back on.

- Martyrdom was saintly for Joan of Arc and the heroines in Victorian novels; in our culture it is a stressor you're better off without. Instead of being overwhelmed by the constant care of infants or invalids, arrange for an occasional surrogate. If sitters or nurses are neither available nor financially feasible, try for a trade-off. One housebound mother of five retains her equilibrium by working two half-days each week in a bookstore while the owner revels in taking over as part-time grandma.

Rather than suffering in silence while stressing yourself out with an unfair workload, admit you aren't Superwoman and ask for assistance. If no one rallies 'round, help yourself—even if it entails requesting a job transfer or foregoing a luxury to pay a weekly cleaning service.

• Hassles (ordinary occurrences that burgeon into stressors) can be manipulated into manageability if tackled on their own turf. For instance: if you're frazzled out before your day's work commences, the cause could be the early-morning hassle of getting your family off to school and work. Having everyone's clothing and accouterments laid out the night before and making bunches of lunches on the weekend (frozen sandwiches self-defrost by lunchtime) avoids the stressful confusion of sewing on a shirt button and searching for a misplaced paper while spreading peanut butter.

An additional hassle might be your daily commute. (The September 1988 *University of California, Berkeley Wellness Letter* reports that each year hundreds of drivers get angry enough to assault offending motorists with deadly weapons—California freeways accounted for 70 such cases in 1987.) Try changing your route or your mode of transportation: form a carpool or withdraw from one; take a bus, ride your bike, walk... do whatever it takes to make the least of your stress and the most of your life. Your good looks and good health are worth it.

How to Relax

Consciously breathing deeply is the opening gambit for all types of deliberate relaxation because it reverses the stress- instigated shallow, rapid respiration that changes blood chemistry. Inhaling for 6 seconds, holding your breath for a count of 3, then exhaling for 6 seconds is a complete-unto-itself stress-reliever when repeated for 2 minutes.

Progressive relaxation

Relaxing on cue requires practice, but once mastered, the stress-relieving relaxation response can be achieved with a few deep breaths. "Progressive Relaxation," based on a 5,000-year-old Yoga tranquility exercise and well publicized by Dr. Herbert Benson, [13, 14, 15] can be varied according to environmental circumstances and personal preferences.

1. Sit or lie in a comfortable position with your eyes closed.
2. Breathe deeply.
3. Tense, then relax each muscle group. Begin with your feet, move up through your legs, torso, arms, neck and face, and concentrate on the feeling of tension sliding away. Some experts recommend starting at the top and working down to your feet, others suggest talking to the different parts of your body, telling them to relax.
4. Remain relaxed while breathing naturally for 5 to 30 minutes. Slowly counting down from 10 to 1 can increase the depth of relaxation. Imagining yourself slowly descending on an escalator past placards bearing numbers from 10 to 1, and telling yourself, "Ten, I am growing more relaxed. Nine, I am growing..." may help achieve relaxation.
5. At the end of your session, saying, "When I count from 1 to 5 I will open my eyes and feel refreshed and energetic," helps produce the desired effects. Before resuming normal activities, blink your eyes, yawn, and stretch.

Using a mantra

There is nothing mystic about a mantra. It need not be a secret incantation assigned by a guru, it can be any sound or word you select as an adjunct to deep breathing and relaxation. Inhale through your nostrils, exhale through your mouth; concentrate on and softly hum the word of your choice.

Meditating

Absence of thought, not profound rumination, is the goal of this form of meditation which reduces the activity of the nervous system. Focusing on a mantra or the words of a brief phrase or prayer helps exclude interference from external distractions. If other thoughts intrude, push them out of your mind and return to your passive repetition.

Visualizing

Imagining yourself in a peacefully pleasant situation can enhance physical and mental relaxation. For the greatest benefit, make your mental imagery detailed and vivid. If you visualize yourself lying on a beach, "see" the blue sky and swaying palm trees, "hear" the cry of a gull and the soothing sound of waves lapping at the shore, "feel" the warmth of the sun and the grittiness of the sand, "smell" the tangy salt air. For a two-minute stress reliever:

1. Lie down, sit comfortably, or stand and lean against a wall. Close your eyes.
2. Tense all your muscles while you inhale deeply for 6 seconds. Let your body go limp while you exhale. Take a few normal breaths, then repeat the sequence.
3. Visualize the word "calm" or imagine a calm, happy scene for about a minute, then open your eyes, yawn and stretch.

Programming your subconscious

Sequestered within every sub-subconscious is an eager-to-please, primordial genie with awesome powers. Aside from attending to autonomic (involuntary) physical functions, it docilely waits to be summoned. When, through relaxation, the confining "stopper" is removed, the genie can be instructed to relieve stress, influence reactions and future behavior, and improve everything from your appearance to your tennis serve. The potential is practically unlimited, but, like man-made computers, Mother Nature's genie must be programmed by conscious thought in terms it can understand. It has been corked up during our eons of mental development, so orders must be issued as simple statements of facts to be accomplished, and illustrated with visualizations of the desired results. However they're labeled (Autogenic Training, Guided Meditation, Psycho-Cybernetics, Psychosynthesis, Scientology, Mind Control, Transcendental Meditation, etc.), here are the basic guidelines for conscious-subconscious communication:

- Use positive statements and images. If you want to stop biting your fingernails, say, "My nails are growing longer and more lovely," while imagining yourself admiring your attractively long-nailed fingers. *Don't* say, "I'm not going to bite my nails any more," and *don't* visualize your raggedy fingertips.

- Concentrate on only one situation per session. For instance: if you have prepared a speech but are uptight over delivering it, table your nail-growing or whatever improvement you have been working on. "Walk" yourself through the presentation at each of several relaxation sessions to establish a "memory" of success that will relieve stressful feelings and make your speech a foregone smash. "See" yourself walking onstage and smiling confidently at the audience, "feel" the lectern as you arrange your notes, "hear" the responsive laughter when you pause after your comic line, and "enjoy" the applause as you return to your seat.

How Exercise Helps to Control Stress

Relaxation is the ideal prophylactic for stress; exercise the perfect antidote. The body is designed to release tension through physical activity which instigates the production of tranquilizing endorphins and burns up the superfluous chemicals, sugars, and fats produced during stress. Chronic stress contracts muscles and deprives them of oxygen, causing them to become tense and painful. Taking a brief "exercise break" can de-stress your muscles and dissipate accumulating stress. Dr. Robert Thayer, of California State University at Long Beach, has found that a brisk ten-minute walk decreases tension and elevates the mood of his subjects for an hour. When you are at work and an outdoor walk isn't feasible, try striding up and down the hall, climbing stairs to the next floor, or executing a few "jumping jacks" in the powder room.

Several studies have shown that people who follow a regular program of aerobic exercise have fewer stress hormones circulating through their systems and have better stress tolerance than their sedentary counterparts. Combining aerobics with relaxation and guided imagery relieves existing stress and provides a defense against future stresses.

1. Perform any aerobic activity to bring your heart rate into its target zone for 1 to 2 minutes.
2. Relax limply and visualize a peaceful scene for 1 to 3 minutes.
3. Repeat the 5-minute cycles of alternating movement and relaxation 6 to 10 times.

Nine Natural Aids for Combating Stress

Swings or hammocks were once prescribed as therapeutic "passive exercise." Rocking in a chair relieves muscular tension and lulls adults as well as infants. Listening to music—peacefully melodic sounds, not toe-tapping rhythms—soothes body and mind. Here are some other natural aids for combating stress.

1. *Approach it positively.* Regarding a partially filled glass as half empty or half full has less to do with stress tolerance than the pessimistic refusal to refill it lest the liquid evaporate or be spilled. Optimists are sometimes proven wrong, but they live longer and enjoy life more.

2. *Call time-out.* The amount and type of personal "down" time required varies with each individual, but we all need some of it. Whether it is an evening to devote to a beautifying facial and bath or an uninterrupted half day to read or pursue a hobby, we must do something for ourselves on frequent occasions. This was the prescription a wise doctor gave one of his patients whose sudden rise in blood pressure was accompanied by an assortment of minor ailments. When queried about what she had been doing, her prideful statement that career and family duties occupied all her waking hours elicited no praise, merely the terse comment, "That could be the problem. Take some time out for yourself and come back in a month. You may not need any medication." She didn't. By delegating a few of her supposedly indispensable chores she "found" time for personal pleasures and was rewarded with a clean bill of health at her next medical checkup.

3. *Care for a pet.* Many studies show that interaction with an animal brings about a decrease in stress reactions. Even aquarium-watching is soothing—witness the proliferation of tension-dispelling fish tanks in doctors' and dentists' offices.

4. *Cry it out.* Emotional tears, not those engendered by dicing onions, carry off harmful stress chemicals.

5. *Laugh it off.* Norman Cousins' book, *Anatomy of an Illness*, established the value of humor in healing. Laughter also relieves tension. Laughing at professional comic routines is great therapy; chuckling at the funny side of our own discomfortures helps keep them in perspective.

6. *Put it into words.* Translating your innermost thoughts into conscious words can blow off steam, reduce worry, and increase stress tolerance. If you are being beset by stressors, write out a description of each one, along with a list of things you can do to modify or abolish it. If you are furious at your boss, compose a letter containing all the caustic comments you've been squelching. Read it over, then tear it up. If you would rather verbalize than put words on paper, turn on your tape recorder, shout out your fury or describe your woes to an imaginary therapist. Play it back, then erase the tape.

7. *Sleep it off.* Sleep is an antidote to stress. It reverses stress-instigated physical changes and helps replenish depleted neuro-

chemicals. How much sleep we need is genetically determined, can vary from 3 to 11 hours out of each 24, decreases as we grow older, and increases when we are under stress. However, wakefulness in times of stress is part of the fight-or- flight survival mechanism and, unless controlled, stress and sleeplessness can create a viciously self-perpetuating cycle that leaves us looking and feeling drained. Sleep experts offer the following tips for encouraging a good night's rest.

- Avoid caffeine-containing beverages for 4 hours before bedtime.

- Unwind by doing something unstressful (read, watch television, take a bath) before preparing for bed.

- Eat a *light* snack: crackers and cheese, a small bowl of cereal and milk, or a scoop of ice cream.

- Drink a cup of warm milk with a spoonful of honey or blackstrap molasses. Or try a soporific herbal tea (blackberry, camomile, catnip, dandelion, hops, lavender flowers, lemon balm, peppermint, red clover, sage, St. Johnswort, valerian). For a potent nightcap: mix 2 tablespoons valerian root with 1 tablespoon *each* lavender flowers, lemon balm, and passion flowers. Steep 1 teaspoon of the herbal mixture in 1 cup hot water for 10 minutes.

- Take a calcium-magnesium supplement, or 100 milligrams of B-5 plus 1,000 milligrams of inositol, or up to 2 grams of tryptophan. Durk Pearson and Sandy Shaw[124] recommend accompanying the tryptophan with 100 milligrams of B-6 and 1,000 milligrams of vitamin C. These natural sleep inducers have been found to be as effective as "sleeping pills," with none of the habit-forming or next-day-hangover residuals of pharmaceuticals. If you are troubled by wakefulness during the night, a report in the May 1988 *Federation Proceedings* suggests increasing the copper and iron in your diet (see Vitamin and Mineral Chart) or taking a mineral supplement.

- Perform a few gentle bending and stretching exercises.

- Practice your progressive relaxation technique after you are in bed. Visualize yourself sleeping peacefully. Implant the suggestion that you are going to drift off into sound sleep, then awaken refreshed at the sound of the alarm.

8. Soak it away. Before being supplanted by drugs, baths were used to quiet violent patients in mental hospitals. Dr. Richard S. Gubner, medical director of Safety Harbor Fitness Center in Florida, recommends 15-minute hot (102 degree) baths. Dr. Jens Henriksen, medical director of the Chattanooga Pain Center in

Tennessee, says body-temperature bathwater is more relaxing. Herbalists suggest adding herbs to increase the benefits (see Chapter 8).

Personal preferences for body-soul pampering are the best guides. One busy career woman combines relaxation and meditation with her morning bath. She fills the tub with very hot water, relaxes and shuts out all thoughts by concentrating on the velvety blackness she visualizes with closed eyes. By the time the cooling water rouses her in 15 to 20 minutes, she is ready to meet the day—stress-free and confident that she can handle whatever happens.

9. *Utilize available assistance.* Sharing stresses with discreet clergy, family members, or friends can resolve many stressful difficulties. If you need help in mastering relaxation and coping techniques, there are classes and seminars on everything from Arica and Biofeedback to Zen Buddhism, and professionally prepared tapes covering all areas of stress control.

Stimulating Stressors That Help Fight Boredom

Stress management entails more than coping with our fight-or-flight response; it includes creating stimulating stressors. This apparent incongruity is explained by the fact that *stress underload* (the psychologists' term for boredom) is itself a negative stress than can lead to the same disorders as stress overload. As we mature, our minds gain the capacity to process ever-increasing amounts of information. If no new challenges are provided, the brain may damage the body just to relieve the monotony, or combat its boredom by egging us on to neglect our jobs, overeat, take drugs, or pick fights with our friends.

Stress-underload remedies are remarkably similar to those for controlling stress overload. Changing routes or modes of transportation provides a positive, challenging stress while diminishing commuting frustrations. Learning to care for the pet you acquired to help you relax is exciting. Joining an aerobics class, establishing exercise routines, perfecting progressive relaxation techniques—all help feed the brain's demands for stimulation.

The "time out for yourself" prescription offers unlimited, ongoing opportunities for adding zest to your life. You can take a class or teach a class, attend a concert, paint a picture, plant a garden, study a foreign language, write a book, join a club or start one. The activity needn't be self-centered—organizing a rummage sale for your favorite charity, reading and writing letters for the visually handicapped, or taking your kids to the zoo are other options. "Success" lies in the fun and fascination of learning and doing; "change" is the name of the game. You may enjoy experimenting with different experiences every few weeks, or you may discover latent talents that lead to a second career or after-retirement income.

Life and its beautifully healthful potential are gifts from Mother Nature. By making the most of what we have been given, we not only improve our outward attractiveness, we also add zestfully happy, productive years to our lives.

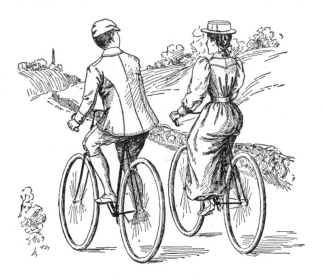

Appendixes

Vitamin & Mineral Chart
Glossary of Key Terms & Ingredients
References
Index

Vitamin and Mineral Chart*

VITAMINS (ingested as foods/supplements)	BENEFITS	
	Beauty	Health
A (retinol, dry or oil based) **Beta carotene** for conversion to A as needed by the body	essential for healthy, moist, skin. Deficiency can cause eruptions or dry, coarse, wrinkled skin; dry hair or dandruff; ridging or peeling fingernails	important for healing, benefits eyes, teeth, mouth, nose and throat linings. Beta carotene is an antioxidant, anti-cancer agent
B COMPLEX (interrelated—a deficiency of one can create a deficiency of all)	essential for healthy skin, hair, and eyes	anti-stress, energizing, and healing. Helps metabolize other nutrients for healthy digestion and nerves
B-1 (thiamine)	important for healthy eyes and hair	helps release energy from carbohydrates; promotes a healthy digestive and nervous system; aids memory and heart function
B-2 (riboflavin—once called vitamin G)	helps eyes, hair, and nails; helps prevent skin dryness and fissures around lips, eye, and mouth corners	same as B complex plus important for respiratory system and vision. Helps prevent fatty deposits on artery walls
B-3 (niacin, nicotinic acid; synthetic, niacinamide or nicotinamide)	helps maintain normal skin function, releases trapped sebum that can create skin problems	same as B complex, natural form may cause flushing by stimulating circulation
B-5 (pantothenic acid, panthenol, or calcium pantothenate)	thickens and repairs damaged hair, with PABA and folic acid helps restore color to gray hair	same as B complex, plus aids B-6 and C in allergy relief, benefits colitis
B-6 (pyridoxine)	helps prevent cracks at mouth corners, skin breakouts, and other stress-related skin problems	aids metabolism of protein and fat, brain function, and formation of red blood cells. Promotes healthy eyes, tongue, and nervous system. Alleviates PMS and "morning sickness"

PRINCIPAL FOOD SOURCES	RDA	TOXICITY unless per MD
dairy products, eggs, green and yellow fruits and vegetables	5,000 IU	50,000 IU for extended periods. Excessive amounts of carotene may yellow skin
brewer's yeast, liver, whole grains	(see individual listings)	excess of one can create a deficiency of the others
same as B complex plus dried legumes; fish; lean beef, pork and poultry; nuts	1.5 mg (more if exercising)	rare
same as B complex plus brussels sprouts, dairy products, and nuts	1.7 mg (more if exercising)	rare
same as B complex plus beef, pork, and poultry; dairy products; nuts, rhubarb, seafood	20 mg	1,000 mg
same as B complex plus kidney, legumes, milk, raw fruits and vegetables, salmon	7 to 15 mg (estimated)	rare
same as B complex plus avocado, banana, beef, cauliflower, chicken, corn, dark leafy greens, eggs, nuts, potatoes, salmon, and tuna	2 to 2.2 mg	rare

Vitamin and Mineral Chart (continued)

VITAMINS (ingested as foods/supplements)	BENEFITS	
	Beauty	Health
B-9 = folic acid, folate, or folacin (once called vitamin M)	delays hair graying when used with B-5 and PABA, promotes healthy skin	acts with B-12 for hemoglobin production. Energizing, promotes healthy nerves
B-12 (cobalamin or cyanocobalamin)	necessary for healthy skin, hair, and nails	anti-anemia; maintains healthy nerves, blood, and tissues
Biotin (co-enzyme R, once called vitamin H)	helps prevent hair loss, premature wrinkles, scaly skin rash	helps circulatory system and release of energy from carbohydrates
Choline	helps maintain healthy hair	aids memory function, lowers cholesterol, soothes nerves. Necessary for storage of vitamin A
Inositol	needed for healthy hair and skin. Helps prevent eczema and falling hair	aids memory function and fat metabolism. Lowers cholesterol
PABA (Para-aminobenzoic acid)	keeps skin smooth and healthy. With B-5 plus folic acid helps restore gray hair	aids blood cell formation and protein utilization. Internal supplements augment sunscreens
VITAMIN C COMPLEX (Ascorbic acid, plus the bioflavonoids—once called vitamin P—citrus flavons, hesperidin, quercetin, and rutin.) Bioflavonoids assist utilization of C and strengthen capillaries. Vitamin C alone, natural or synthetic, is a cold remedy.	regulates sebaceous glands to keep skin from drying out. Helps prevent facial lines, wrinkles and spider veins; hair tangling or breaking	essential for collagen synthesis, healthy bones and cartilage. Promotes healthy eyes, gums, and teeth; helps heal wounds and repair damaged cells. Burned up by stress and tobacco use

PRINCIPAL FOOD SOURCES	RDA	TOXICITY unless per MD
same as B complex plus dairy products, leafy greens, orange juice, oysters, salmon, and tuna	400 to 600 mcg	rare
animal foods	3 to 6 mcg	rare
same as B complex plus dried legumes, egg yolk, kidney, milk, most fresh vegetables, nuts	300 mcg (estimated)	rare
same as B complex plus egg yolk, leafy greens, lecithin supplements, legumes, nuts	none established	rare
same as B complex plus blackstrap molasses, citrus fruit, lecithin supplements, lima beans, milk, nuts	none established	rare
bran, brewer's yeast, molasses, organ meats, unpolished rice, wheat germ, whole grains	none established	rare (excess may cause nausea)
citrus fruits (with white membrane for flavons); broccoli; cabbage; cantaloupe; green peppers; kiwi, strawberries and other fruits; potatoes; raw, leafy greens; tomatoes. (Black currants, blackberries, buckwheat, cherries, and grapes for bioflavonoids.)	60 mg C (Ratio of 5 to 1 for ascorbic acid to bioflavonoids)	rare (excess may cause temporary diarrhea, burning urine, or itchy skin)

Vitamin and Mineral Chart (continued)

VITAMINS (ingested as foods/supplements)	BENEFITS	
	Beauty	Health
D (calciferol, ergosterol, or viosterol)	promotes healthy eyes, skin, and teeth	aids absorption of calcium for healthy bones and nervous system. Best utilized when taken with vitamin A
E (tocopherol, alpha or 7 mixed; dl = synthetic)	helps form muscles and tissues to prevent wrinkles and premature aging of the skin. Helps prevent dry, dull, or falling hair	antioxidant to protect essential fatty acids and cells from destruction. Vasodilator, energizer, and anticoagulant
K (K-1 and K-2 are synthesized by the body, K-3 is chemically manufactured)	helps prevent bruising and premature aging of the skin	helps maintain bone metabolism, reduces excessive menstrual flow, necessary for blood clotting. Vitality and longevity factor

MINERALS (ingested as foods/supplements)	BENEFITS	
	Beauty	Health
CALCIUM (carbonate, gluconate, lactate, orate, tricalcium phosphate—balance with twice as much phosphorus and half as much magnesium; accompany by vitamins A, C, and D)	helps clear blemished skin and revitalize lifeless, tired-looking skin	strengthens bones and teeth, calms tense nerves, helps regulate heart beat and muscle contractions
CHROMIUM (accompany supplements with brewer's yeast to increase absorption)	improves circulation for healthy skin and hair	helps maintain blood sugar level; activates enzymes for carbohydrate, fat and protein metabolism

PRINCIPAL FOOD SOURCES	RDA	TOXICITY unless per MD
fortified milk, beef liver, salmon, and tuna. Produced by the body from the action of sunlight on the skin. Synthetic D manufactured from fish liver oils	400 IU	excess stored in the liver but less toxic than excess vitamin A
asparagus, broccoli, brussels sprouts, butter, dried legumes, egg yolks, leafy greens, liver, olives, soybeans, sunflower seeds, vegetable oils, wheat germ, whole grains	10 to 30 IU	nontoxic under normal conditions. Check with doctor if have high blood pressure, diabetes, or overactive thyroid
egg yolk, fish liver oils, leafy greens, lentils, raw cauliflower, safflower and sunflower oils, yogurt	140 to 500 mcg (estimated)	500 mg of synthetic

PRINCIPAL FOOD SOURCES	RDA	TOXICITY unless per MD
dairy products, dark leafy greens, dried legumes, peanuts, salmon, sardines, shellfish, soybeans, sunflower seeds, walnuts	800 to 1,500 mg	over 2,000 mg may cause drowsiness or calcium deposits in soft tissues
brewer's yeast, cheese, clams, corn oil, liver, meat, whole grains	200 mcg (estimated)	rare

Vitamin and Mineral Chart (continued)

MINERALS (ingested as foods/supplements)	BENEFITS	
	Beauty	Health
COPPER	helps prevent hair-color loss, pale or blotchy skin, and easy bruising	necessary for formation of bones, connective tissues, and red blood cells. Assists healing and normal functions of brain and nervous system
FLUORINE— FLUORIDE (calcium fluoride, synthetic sodium fluoride)		helps prevent tooth decay and osteoporosis. Strengthens bones
IODINE (iodide)	promotes healthy hair, nails, skin, and teeth	energizes, helps thyroid burn excess fat, improves mental alacrity, prevents goiter and hypothyroidism
IRON (ferrous citrate, ferrous fumarate, ferrous gluconate, and ferrous peptonate)	essential for healthy nails, skin color, and hair growth	builds red blood cells to prevent iron-deficiency anemia. Bolsters energy and disease resistance, helps offset stress
MAGNESIUM	prevents skin disorders	helps metabolize calcium, C, and carbohydrates; promotes healthy teeth, nerves, and muscles; energizes, and fights depression
MANGANESE	helps maintain healthy hair	assists utilization of B-1, biotin, C, and E. Aids nervous system and thyroid gland function. Energizes, helps memory and is needed for normal bone and tendon structure

PRINCIPAL FOOD SOURCES	RDA	TOXICITY unless per MD
beef and pork liver, chicken, leafy greens, mushrooms, nuts, raisins, shellfish (especially oysters), whole grains	2 to 4 mg (estimated)	rare
fluoridated drinking water. Traces in gelatin, seafood, tea, and whole grains	4 mg (estimated)	excess can cause mottled teeth, osteoclerosis, and calcification of soft tissues
iodized salt, kelp, onions, seafood, vegetable oils	150 mcg	rare from natural sources, excess supplements can trigger thyroid dysfunction
egg yolks, blackstrap molasses, dark leafy greens, dried fruits and legumes, lean meat, liver, whole wheat	18 mg	rare from natural sources. Supplement only under medical supervision
almonds, apples, apricots, bananas, bran, corn, dairy products, figs, grapefruit and lemons, meats, raw leafy greens, soybeans	300 to 400 mg	can be toxic if not balanced with calcium and phosphorus
bananas, beets, bran, coffee, egg yolks, leafy greens, legumes, nuts, pineapple, tea, and whole grains	2 to 7 mg (estimated)	rare

Vitamin and Mineral Chart (continued)

MINERALS (ingested as foods/supplements)	BENEFITS	
	Beauty	Health
PHOSPHORUS (must be balanced with calcium in order to function)	promotes healthy teeth and gums	aids bone and cell growth and repair; carbohydrate and fat metabolism; energizes
POTASSIUM	helps maintain healthy skin and prevent puffiness	controls fluid balance in tissues; aids mental alacrity and muscle strength; helps regulate blood pressure and heart rhythm, has tranquilizing effect
SELENIUM	maintains skin elasticity, helps prevent and correct dandruff	alleviates menopausal distress; complements vitamin E to prevent cell damage by oxygen
SULFUR	helps maintain healthy hair, nails, and skin. Helps prevent dermatitis, eczema, and psoriasis	facilitates collagen synthesis and tissue formation
ZINC	helps prevent hair loss, brittle or spotted nails; aids formation of collagen to prevent wrinkles; improves acne conditions	essential for protein synthesis and brain function. Important for healing; sense of taste and smell

*This table is not intended to be used for diagnostic or prescriptive purposes. For any diagnosis or treatment of illness, please see your physician. The RDAs shown for some nutrients reflect the results of current studies by the Food and Drug Administration and are higher than those previously published.

PRINCIPAL FOOD SOURCES	RDA	TOXICITY unless per MD
dairy products, dried legumes, egg yolks, fish, poultry, meats, and grains	800 to 1,200 mg	excess reduces calcium absorption
bananas, citrus and dried fruits, coffee, fresh vegetables, kiwi fruit, lean meats, legumes, peanuts, potatoes, tea	1,500 to 6,000 mg (should equal sodium consumed)	excess of supplements can cause muscle weakness and heart disturbance
asparagus, bran, broccoli, chicken, egg yolks, milk, onions, red meat, seafood, tomatoes, whole grains	200 mcg (estimated)	rare
bran, brussels sprouts, cabbage, cheese, clams, eggs, fish, mushrooms, nuts, peas and beans, wheat germ	not established	rare
brewer's yeast, eggs, lean red meat, legumes, mushrooms, nonfat dry milk, pumpkin and sunflower seeds, shellfish (especially oysters), spinach, whole grains	15 mg (estimated)	150 mg from supplements

Glossary of
Key Terms
and Ingredients

almond meal: blanched, pulverized almonds. Available in health food stores or can be made in an electric blender or food processor. (To blanch: bring shelled almonds to a boil in water to cover. Let stand until cool. Drain. Remove skins.) Used for facial scrubs and as an ingredient in many skin-care products.

aloe vera: a plant used since Biblical times to treat burns and skin damage, and condition hair. Easily grown indoors or out, or available as a bottled gel from health food stores.

alum: crystalline potassium-aluminum sold in supermarkets, primarily for pickling. As a cosmetic ingredient it refines pores and tightens skin.

astringent: a liquid, usually containing either alcohol or acetone. Used after cleansing to remove excess oil or makeup residue, tighten pores, restore pH balance, and inhibit the growth of bacteria.

benzoin: a fragrant resin first used as a temple incense in Sumatra; now available from pharmacies as tincture of benzoin. It serves as a preservative and skin toner in natural beauty products.

borax: a mineral containing magnesium chloride. Used in natural beauty products for over a century; now sold in supermarkets as Boraxo.

brewer's yeast: originally a brewing byproduct, now grown on molasses for a food supplement. Used externally to activate circulation, chase wrinkles, and tighten pores.

cocoa butter: (or *oil theobroma*), obtained by separating the fat from the cacao beans used for chocolate; has been a favored skin softener for hundreds of years.

comedones: *whiteheads* (closed comedones) are underskin bumps of trapped sebum. *Blackheads* (open comedones) form when the pores become so clogged they burst and the sebum oxidizes in the air to turn black.

emollient or moisturizer: a substance which locks in moisture to keep the surface of the skin soft and supple.

epidermabrasion: sloughing off of dead skin cells by means of friction or exfoliant substances.

epsom salt: magnesium sulfate, marketed as a cathartic or pain-relieving soak. May be used half-and-half with table salt to equal sea salt in homemade beauty products.

exfoliant or scrub: sloughs dead cells from the skin's surface.

glycerin: a byproduct of soap manufacture available from pharmacies. Long used as a humecant to soften skin by drawing moisture and preventing its evaporation, it also keeps cosmetic products moist and makes them spread more easily.

humecants: water-loving compounds that latch on to moisture and help hold it on the skin's surface.

kelp: mineral-rich seaweed available as granules or powder from health food stores. Used as a salt substitute and as a beauty-product enhancer.

keratolytic: skin peeling agent.

lanolin: a fatty substance obtained from sheep's wool. Used in commercial cosmetics and available from pharmacies—test before using if you are allergic to wool.

lecithin: a natural emulsifier made from soybeans. Available in capsules, granules, liquid, or powder for internal or external use.

loofah: the fibers of a special type of gourd formed into friction gloves, bath mitts, or sponges. When lightly rubbed over the body, a loofah stimulates circulation and carries away dead cells and debris.

mayonnaise: commercially bottled or homemade, it is excellent for skin or hair. Cosmetic mayonnaise may be made by omitting the seasonings from any standard recipe, or made in an electric blender from these room-temperature ingredients:

1 whole egg

1 teaspoon honey

1-1/4 cups vegetable or nut oil

3 tablespoons fresh lemon juice

Whir egg, honey, and 1/4 cup oil until combined. With blender running, slowly add 1/2 cup oil, then the lemon juice, then the remaining oil. Blend until thickened; store in the refrigerator.

mineral water: marketed as a bubbly beverage, the trace minerals it contains are absorbed by and benefit the skin when applied as a skin freshener or as an ingredient of other natural beauty products.

occlusive: an oil, cream, or lotion applied as a protective film to trap moisture and prevent its evaporation from the surface of the skin; and to prevent contaminants from makeup or airborne pollutants from seeping into the skin (See also emollient).

papules and pustules: inflamed, pus-filled bumps on the skin's surface resulting from an under-skin infection and the body's defensive effort of sending white blood cells to the area.

petroleum jelly: a derivative of petroleum, once called *petrolatum*, now marketed as Vaseline.

pH: the pH scale (0 to 14) shows the acid/alkaline balance: 0 to 6.9 indicates acidity, 7.0 is neutral, 7.1 or above is alkaline. Contact with an alkaline substance such as soap necessitates an acid-containing toner to restore the healthy skin and hair balance of between pH 3.0 and pH 5.5.

sebum: a combination of oil and wax carried to the skin surface by the sebaceous glands.

toner: an acid-containing liquid used as a skin freshener or astringent to restore a normal pH balance.

white vegetable shortening: vegetable oils hydrogenated into a creamy solid that can be used as a makeup remover or beauty-product ingredient. Marketed as Crisco.

witch hazel: a liquid commercially extracted with alcohol from the bark and leaves of the witch hazel shrub for use as a mild antiseptic and astringent. Also available as a dry herb.

References

1. Adams, Rex. *Miracle Medicine Foods*. West Nyack, NY: Parker Publishing Company, Inc., 1977.

2. Aero, Rita. *The Complete Book of Longevity*. New York: Perigee Books, 1980.

3. Albrecht, Karl. *Stress and the Manager*. Englewood Cliffs, NJ: Prentice-Hall, Inc., 1979.

4. Allen, Oliver E., and editors of Time-Life Books. *Building Sound Bones and Muscles*. Alexandria, VA: Library of Health/Time-Life Books, 1981.

5. Arnold, Caroline. *Too Fat? Too Thin? Do You Have a Choice?* New York: William Morrow and Company, 1984.

6. Arpel, Adrien, with Ronnie Sue Ebenstein. *Adrien Arpel's 3-Week CRASH Makeover/Shapeover Beauty Program*. New York: Rawson Associates Publishers, Inc., 1977.

7. ———. *How to Look Ten Years Younger*. New York: Rawson, Wade Publishers, Inc., 1980.

8. Atkinson, Holly, M.D. *Women and Fatigue*. New York: Putnam's Sons, 1986.

241

9. Bailey, Adrian. *The Blessings of Bread*. New York: Paddington Press Ltd., 1975.

10. Bailey, Covert. *Fit or Fat?*. Boston: Houghton Mifflin Company, 1978.

11. Beeton, Mrs. Isabella. *Beeton's Book of Household Management*. London: S.O. Beeton, 1861.

12. Begoun, Paula. *Blue Eyeshadow Should Be Illegal*. 2nd edition. Seattle, WA: Beginning Press, 1986.

13. Benson, Herbert, M.S. *Beyond the Relaxation Response*. New York: Times Books, 1984.

14. ———. *The Relaxation Response*. New York: William Morrow and Company, Inc., 1975.

15. ———. *Your Maximum Mind*. New York: Times Books, 1987.

16. Bernhardt, Dr. Roger and David Martin. *Self-Mastery Through Self-Hypnosis*. Indianapolis/New York: Bobbs-Merrill Company, Inc., 1977.

17. Birnes, Nancy. *Cheaper and Better*. New York: Harper & Row, Publishers, 1987.

18. Bland, Jeffery. *Medical Applications of Clinical Nutrition*. New Canaan, CT: Keats Publishing Co., 1983.

19. Blaurock-Busch, Eleanor, Ph.D., with Bernd W. Busch, D.C. *The No-Drugs Guide to Better Health*. West Nyack, NY: Parker Publishing Company, Inc., 1984.

20. Bloomfield, Harold H., M.D., and Robert B. Kory. *Happiness*. New York: Simon & Schuster, 1976.

21. Brenton, Myron. *Aging Slowly*. Emmaus, PA: Rodale Press, Inc., 1983.

22. Bricklin, Mark. *The Practical Encyclopedia of Natural Healing*. Emmaus, PA: Rodale Press, Inc., 1976.

23. ———. *Rodale's Encyclopedia of Natural Home Remedies*. Emmaus, PA: Rodale Press, Inc., 1982.

24. Bricklin, Mark, editor. *The Natural Healing Annual, 1986*. Emmaus, PA: Rodale Press, Inc., 1986.

25. ———. *The Natural Healing Annual, 1987*. Emmaus, PA: Rodale Press, Inc., 1987.

26. ———. *The Natural Healing Annual, 1988*. Emmaus, PA: Rodale Press, Inc., 1988.

27. Briggs, George M., and Doris H. Calloway. *Bogert's Nutrition and Physical Fitness.* 11th edition. New York: Holt, Rinehart and Winston Co., 1984.

28. Brody, Jane E. *Jane Brody's Nutrition Book.* New York: Bantam Books, Inc., 1982.

29. Cameron, Myra. *Treasury of Home Remedies.* Englewood Cliffs, NJ: Prentice-Hall, Inc. 1987.

30. Campbell, Greg. *The Joy of Jumping.* New York: Richard Marek Publishers, 1978.

31. Carroll, David. *The Complete Book of Natural Medicines.* New York: Summit Books, 1980.

32. Castleton, Virginia. *The Handbook of Natural Beauty.* Emmaus, PA: Rodale Press, Inc., 1975.

33. Chang, Dr. Stephen T. *The Complete System of Self- Healing.* San Francisco, CA: Tao Publishing, 1986.

34. Chang, Edward C., Ph.D., translator. *Knocking at the Gate of Life and Other Healing Exercises from China.* Emmaus, PA: Rodale Press, 1985.

35. Chase, A.W., M.D. *Dr. Chase's Recipes; or Information for Everybody.* Ann Arbor, MI: Published by the author, 1863; 1866 editions.

36. Chenault, Alice A. *Nutrition and Health.* New York: Holt, Rinehart and Winston Co., 1984.

37. Child, Mrs. Lydia Marie. *The American Frugal Housewife.* Boston: American Stationers' Company, 1836.

38. Clark, Linda. *Face Improvement Through Exercise and Nutrition.* New Canaan, CT: Keats Publishing, Inc., 1970.

39. ———. *Handbook of Natural Remedies for Common Ailments.* Greenwich, CT: Devon-Adair Company, 1976.

40. ———. *Secrets of Health and Beauty.* New York: Pyramid Books, 1974.

41. ———. *Stay Young Longer.* New York: Devon-Adair Company, 1962.

42. Connor, Sonja L., M.S., R.D. and William E. Connor, M.D. *The New American Diet.* New York: Simon & Schuster, 1986.

43. Consumer Guide Editors. *Flatten Your Stomach.* New York: Beekman House, 1979.

44. Craig, Marjorie. *Miss Craig's 21-Day Shape-Up Program.* New York: Random House, 1968.

45. Crenshaw, Mary Ann. *The Natural Way to Super Beauty*. New York: Dell Publishing Co., Inc., 1974.

46. Cross, Jean. *In Grandmother's Day*. Englewood Cliffs, NJ: Prentice-Hall, 1980.

47. Daché, Lilly. *Lilly Daché's Glamour Book*. Philadelphia and New York: J. B. Lippincott Company, 1956.

48. Davis, Adelle. *Let's Eat Right to Keep Fit*. New York: Harcourt Brace Javanovich, Inc., 1970 revised edition.

49. ———. *Let's Get Well*. New York: Harcourt Brace Javanovich, Inc., 1965.

50. Davis, Phyllis B. *Looking Good, Feeling Beautiful*. New York: Simon & Schuster/Avon Products, Inc., 1981.

51. DeBakey, Michael E., M.D. *The Living Heart Diet*. New York: Simon & Schuster, 1984.

52. Dick, William B. *Dick's Encyclopedia of Practical Receipts and Processes or How They Did It in the 1870's*. New York: Funk & Wagnalls, reprint edition prepared by Leicester and Harriet Handsfield.

53. Eaton, S. Boyd, M.D., Marjorie Shostak and Melvin Konnor, M.D., Ph.D. *The Paleolithic Prescription: A Program of Diet & Exercise and a Design for Living*. New York: Harper & Row, 1988.

54. Edelstein, Barbara, M.D. *The Underburner's Diet*. New York: Macmillan Publishing Company, 1987.

55. Faelten, Sharon, David Diamond & the editors of Prevention Magazine. *Take Control of Your Life*. Emmaus, PA: Rodale Press, 1988.

56. Failes, Janice McCall, and Frank W. Cawood. *Natural Healing Encyclopedia*. Peachtree City, GA: FC&A Publishing, 1987.

57. Ferri, Elisa, with Mary-Ellen Siegel. *Finger Tips*. New York: Clarkson N. Potter, Inc./Publishers, 1988.

58. Fitzgibbon, Theodora. *The Food of the Western World*. New York: Quadrangle/The New York Times Book Co., 1976.

59. Frank, Dr. Benjamin S.*Nucleic Acid Therapy in Aging and Degenerative Disease*. New York: Psychological Library, 1974 revised edition.

60. Franklyn, Robert A., M.D., and Marcia Borie. *A Doctor's Quick Way to Achieve Lasting Beauty*. New York: Information Incorporated, 1970.

61. Fredericks, Carleton. *Eat Well, Get Well, Stay Well*. New York: Grosset & Dunlap, 1980.

62. Fredericks, Carleton, and Herbert Bailey. *Food Facts and Fallacies.* New York: Arco Publishing Company, Inc., 1978.

63. Gardner, Joseph L., editor.*Eat Better, Live Better.* Pleasantville, NY: The Reader's Digest Association, Inc., 1982.

64. Garrison, Robert H., and Elizabeth Somer. *The Nutrition Desk Reference.* New Canaan, CT: Keats Publishing Co., 1985.

65. Gilmore, C. P. *Exercising for Fitness.* Alexandria, VA: Library of Health/Time-Life Books, 1981.

66. Goldbeck, Nikki and David. *The Dieter's Companion.* New York: Signet, 1977.

67. Goodenough, Josephus, M.D. *Dr. Goodenough's Home Cures and Herbal Remedies.* (Revised edition of *The Favorite Medical Receipt Book and Home Doctor,* 1904) New York: Avenel Books, 1982.

68. Goodman, Harriet Wilinsky, and Barbara Morse. *Just What the Doctor Ordered.* New York: Holt, Rinehart and Winston, 1982.

69. Grossbart, Ted, Ph.D., and Carl Sherman. *Skin Deep: A Mind/Body Program for Healthy Skin.* New York: William Morrow & Co., Inc., 1985.

70. Guinness, Alma E., editor. *ABC's of the Human Body.* Pleasantville, NY: The Reader's Digest Association, Inc., 1987.

71. Hamilton, Eva M., and Elinor N. Whitney. *Understanding Nutrition.* 4th edition. St. Paul, MN: West Publishing Co., 1984.

72. Harris, Ben Charles. *The Compleat Herbal.* New York: Larchmont, 1972.

73. ———. *Kitchen Medicines.* New York: Weathervane Books, 1968 edition.

74. Hauser, Gayelord. *Gayelord Hauser's Treasury of Secrets.* New York: Farrar, Straus and Company, 1963.

75. ———. *Look Younger, Live Longer.* New York: Fawcett World Library, 1971 revised edition.

76. Heimlich, Henry J., M.D., with Lawrence Galton. *Dr. Heimlich's Home Guide to Emergency Medical Situations.* New York: Simon & Schuster, 1980.

77. Hill, Ann, editor. *A Visual Encyclopedia of Unconventional Medicine.* New York: Crown Publishers Inc., 1979.

78. Hirschhorn, Howard H. *Pain-Free Living: How to Prevent and Eliminate Pain All Over the Body.* West Nyack, NY: Parker Publishing Company, Inc., 1977.

79. Holistic Health Center staff. *The Holistic Health Handbook*. Berkeley, CA: And/Or Press, 1978.

80. Hupping, Carol, Cheryl Winters Tetreau, and Roger B. Yepsen, Jr., editors. *Hints, Tips and Everyday Wisdom*. Emmaus, PA: Rodale Press, Inc., 1985.

81. Hutchinson, E. *Ladies' Indispensable Assistant*. New York: Published by the author, 1852.

82. Imber, Gerald, M.D., and Stephen Brill Kurtin, M.D. *Face Care*. New York: A & W Publishers, Inc., 1983.

83. Jackson, Carole. *Color Me Beautiful*. New York: Ballantine Books, 1981 edition.

84. Jarvis, D.C., M.D. *Folk Medicine*. New York: Henry Holt & Co., Inc., 1958.

85. Kingsley, Philip. *The Complete Hair Book*. New York: Grosset & Dunlap, 1979.

86. Kirschmann, John D. *Nutrition Almanac*. New York: McGraw-Hill, 1979 revised edition.

87. Kloss, Jethro. *Back to Eden*. Santa Barbara, CA: Woodbridge Press Publishing Company, 1975.

88. Korth, Leslie O., D.O., M.R.O. *Some Unusual Healing Methods*. Surrey, England: Health Science Press, 1960.

89. Kounovsky, Nicholas. *Instant Fitness*. New York: Paragon Books, 1979.

90. ———. *The Joy of Feeling Fit*. New York: E. P. Dutton & Co., Inc., 1971.

91. Lamb, Lawrence E., M.D. *What You Need to Know About Food & Cooking for Health*. New York: The Viking Press, 1973.

92. Lawrence, Herbert, M.D. *The Care of Your Skin*. New York: Gramercy Publishing Company, 1955.

93. Lawson, Donna. *Looking Fit & Fabulous at Forty Plus*. Emmaus, PA: Rodale Press, 1987.

94. Lesser, Gershon M., M.D. *Growing Younger*. New York: St. Martin's Press, 1987.

95. Leyel, Mrs. C. F. *Herbal Delights*. New York: Gramercy Publishing Company, 1986.

96. Lillyquist, Michael J. *Sunlight and Health*. New York: Dodd Mead & Co., 1985.

97. Loewenfeld, Claire, and Philippa Back. *Herbs, Health and Cookery*. New York: Gramercy Publishing Company, 1965.

98. Lubowe, Irwin I., M.D. *New Hope for Your Skin*. New York: E. P. Dutton, 1963.

99. Lucas, Richard. *Nature's Medicines*. West Nyack, NY: Parker Publishing Company, Inc., 1966.

100. Maltz, Maxwell, M.D., F.I.C.S. *Psycho-Cybernetics*. Englewood Cliffs, NJ: Prentice-Hall, Inc., 1960.

101. McDougall, John A., M.D., and Mary A. McDougall. *The McDougall Plan*. Piscataway, NJ: New Century Publishers, Inc., 1983.

102. McKee, Alma. *To Set Before a Queen*. New York: Simon & Schuster, 1964.

103. Meyer, Clarence. *American Folk Medicine*. New York: New American Library, 1973.

104. ———. *Vegetarian Medicines*. Glenwood, IL: Meyerbooks, 1981.

105. Miller, Fred D., D.D.S. *Open Door to Health*. New York: The Devon-Adair Co., 1959.

106. Miller, Peter M., Dr. *The Hilton Head Metabolism Diet*. New York: Warner Books, Inc., 1983.

107. Mindell, Earl. *Earl Mindell's Quick and Easy Guide to Better Health*. New Canaan, CT: Keats Publishing, Inc., 1982.

108. ———. *Earl Mindell's Shaping Up with Vitamins*. New York: Warner Books, Inc., 1985.

109. ———. *Earl Mindell's Vitamin Bible*. New York: Warner Books, 1979.

110. Mitchell, Curtis. *The Perfect Exercise: The Hop, Skip and Jump Way to Health*. New York: Simon & Schuster, Inc., 1976.

111. Morris, Freda. *Self-Hypnosis in Two Days*. New York: E.P. Dutton & Co., 1975.

112. Morrison, Marsh, D.C., Ph.C., F.I.C.C. *Doctor Morrison's Miracle Guide to Pain-Free Health and Longevity*. West Nyack, NY: Parker Publishing Company, Inc., 1977.

113. Murphy, Wendy, and editors of Time-Life Books. *Touch, Taste, Smell, Sight and Hearing*. Alexandria, VA: Library of Health/Time-Life Books, 1982.

114. Nagler, Willibald, M.D. *Dr. Nagler's Body Maintenance and Repair Book*. New York: Simon & Schuster, 1987.

115. Norfolk, Dr. Donald. *The Habits of Health*. New York: St. Martin's Press, 1976.

116. Notelovitz, Morris, with Marsha Ware. *Stand Tall! The Informed Woman's Guide to Preventing Osteoporosis.* Gainesville, FL: Triad Publishing Company, 1982.

117. Nudel, Adele. *For the Woman Over 50.* New York: Avon books, 1979.

118. Null, Gary and Steve. *Complete Handbook of Nutrition.* New York: Dell Publishing Co., Inc., 1972.

119. Osmond, Marie, with Julie Davis. *Marie Osmond's Guide to Beauty, Health, and Style.* New York: Simon & Schuster, 1980.

120. Palm, J. Daniel, Ph.D. *Diet Away Your Stress, Tension, and Anxiety.* New York: Pocket Books, 1976.

121. Parrish, John A., Barbara A. Gilchrist, Thomas B. Fitzpatrick. *Between You and Me.* Boston: Little, Brown, 1978.

122. Pauling, Linus. *How to Live Longer and Feel Better.* New York: W. H. Freeman and Company, 1986.

123. Pearson, Dr. Leonard, Lillian R. Pearson, M.S.W., and Karola Saekel. *The Psychologist's Sensational Cookbook.* New York: Peter H. Wyden Publisher, 1974.

124. Pearson, Durk, and Sandy Shaw. *Life Extension.* New York: Warner Books, 1983.

125. People's Medical Publishing House Staff. *The Chinese Way to a Long and Healthy Life.* New York: Bell Publishing Company, 1987

126. Petulengro, Leon. *The Roots of Health.* New York: New American Library, 1968.

127. Pfeiffer, Carl C. *Zinc and Other Micro-Nutrients.* New Canaan, CT: Keats Publishing Co., 1978.

128. Pinkham, Mary Ellen. *How to Become a Healthier, Prettier You.* Garden City, NY: Doubleday & Company, Inc., 1984.

129. Prevention Magazine editors. *The Complete Book of Vitamins.* Emmaus, PA: Rodale Press, 1984.

130. ———. *The Encyclopedia of Common Diseases.* Emmaus, PA: Rodale Press, 1976.

131. ———. *Herbs for Health.* Emmaus, PA: Rodale Press, 1979.

132. ———. *The Natural Way to a Healthy Skin.* Emmaus, PA: Rodale Press, 1972.

133. Principal, Victoria. *The Beauty Principal.* New York: Simon & Schuster, 1984.

134. Prudden, Bonnie. *Bonnie Prudden's Fitness Book*. New York: The Ronald Press Company, 1959.

135. Pugh, Katie. *Baldness: Is It Necessary?* Richmond, VA: Mailing Services, Inc., 1967.

136. Randolph, Vance. *Ozark Magic & Folklore*. New York: Dover Publications, Inc., 1964.

137. Registein, Quentin, M.D. *Sound Sleep*. New York: Simon & Schuster, 1980.

138. Reilly, Harold H. and Ruth Hagy Brod. *The Edgar Cayce Handbook for Health Through Drugless Therapy*. New York: Macmillan Publishing Company, 1975.

139. Riedman, Sarah. *The Good Looks Skin Book*. New York: Julian Messner, 1983.

140. Rose, Jeanne. *Herbs and Things*. New York: Grosset & Dunlap, 1972.

141. Rodale, J.I. and Staff. *The Complete Book of Minerals for Health*. Emmaus, PA: Rodale Books, Inc., 1972.

142. Rossiter, Frederick M., M.D. *Face Culture*. New York: Pageant Books, Inc., 1956.

143. Roth, Beulah. *The International Beauty Book*. Los Angeles: Price/Stern/Sloan Publishers, 1970.

144. Royal, Penny C. *Herbally Yours*. Payson, UT: Sound Nutrition, 1982.

145. Rutledge, Deborah. *Natural Beauty Secrets*. New York: Hawthorne Books, 1966.

146. Saffon, M.J. *The 15-Minute-A-Day Natural Face Lift*. Englewood Cliffs, NJ: Prentice-Hall Inc., 1979.

147. Sassoon, Beverly and Vidal, with Camille Duhe. *A Year of Beauty and Health*. New York: Simon & Schuster, 1978.

148. Saunders, Rubie. *The Beauty Book*. New York: Julian Messner, 1983.

149. Schoen, Linda Allen, editor. *AMA Book of Skin and Hair Care*. Philadelphia, PA: J.B. Lippincott Company, 1976.

150. Schorr, Lia. *Lia Schorr's Skin Care Guide for Men*. Englewood Cliffs, NJ: Prentice-Hall, Inc., 1985.

151. Schurmann, Petra. *Be Beautiful!* Tucson, AZ: H P Books, Fisher Publishing Inc., 1984.

152. Schwartz, Alice Kuhn, Ph.D. and Norma S. Aaron. *Somniquest*. New York: Harmony Books, 1979.

153. Sehnert, Keith W., M.D., with Howard Eisenberg. *How to Be Your Own Doctor (Sometimes)*. New York: Grosset & Dunlap, 1981.

154. Selye, Hans, M.D. *The Stress of Life*. New York: McGraw-Hill Book Company, Inc., 1956.

155. Shames, Richard, M.D. and Chuck Sterin, M.S., Ph.D. *Healing with Mind Power*. Emmaus, PA: Rodale Press, 1978.

156. Shute, Evan V. *Common Questions on Vitamin E and Their Answers*. New Canaan, CT: Keats Publishing Co., 1979.

157. Shute, Wilfrid E. *Health Preserver*. Emmaus, PA: Rodale Press, 1977.

158. Siegel, Bernie S., M.D. *Love, Medicine and Miracles*. New York: Harper & Row, Publishers, 1986.

159. Smith, Ann. *Celebrity Exercise*. New York: Walker and Company, 1976.

160. Soglow, M. H. *Relax Your Way to Health*. Englewood Cliffs, NJ: Prentice-Hall, 1958.

161. Stabile, Toni. *Cosmetics: The Great American Skin Game*. New York: Ballantine Books, 1973.

162. Stein, Laura. *The Bloomingdale's Eat Healthy Diet*. New York: St. Martin's Press, 1986.

163. Sternberg, Thomas H., M.D. *More Than Skin Deep*. New York: Doubleday & Co., Inc., 1970.

164. Swarth, Judith. *Skin, Hair, Nails, and Nutrition*. San Diego, CA: Health Media of America, Inc., 1986.

165. Tannahill, Reay. *Food in History*. New York: Stein and Day/Publishers, 1973.

166. Tapley, Donald F., M.D., Robert J. Weiss, M.D., and Thomas Q. Morris, M.D., medical editors. *Complete Home Medical Guide*. New York: Crown Publishers, Inc., 1985.

167. Thomas, Mai. *Grannies' Remedies*. New York: Gramercy Publishing Company, 1965.

168. Time-Life Books consultants. *Eating Right*. Alexandria, VA: Time-Life Books Inc., 1987.

169. ———. *The Fit Body*. Alexandria, VA: Time-Life Books Inc., 1987.

170. ———. *Getting Firm*. Alexandria, VA: Time-Life Books Inc., 1987.

171. ———. *Managing Stress*. Alexandria, VA: Time-Life Books Inc., 1987.

172. ———. *Restoring the Body*. Alexandria, VA: Time-Life Books Inc., 1987.

173. ———. *Staying Flexible*. Alexandria, VA: Time-Life Books Inc., 1987.

174. ———. *Wholesome Diet*. Alexandria, VA: Library of Health/Time-Life Books Inc., 1981.

175. Van Fleet, James K., D.C. *Extraordinary Healing Secrets from a Doctor's Private Files*. West Nyack, NY: Parker Publishing Company, Inc., 1977.

176. Vaughan, Beatrice. *The Old Cook's Almanac*. New York: Gramercy Publishing Company, 1966.

177. Veyne, Paul, editor. *A History of Private Life*. Cambridge, MA: The Belknap Press of Harvard University Press, 1987.

178. Wade, Carlson. *Health Secrets from the Orient*. West Nyack, NY: Parker Publishing Company, Inc., 1973.

179. ———. *Helping Yourself with New Enzyme Catalyst Health Secrets*. West Nyack, NY: Parker Publishing Company, Inc., 1981.

180. ———. *Natural Folk Remedies*. Greenwich, CT: Globe Communications Corp., 1979.

181. Wagonvoord, James, editor. *The Man's Book*. New York: Avon Books, 1978.

182. Weiner, Michael A., Ph.D., and Kathleen Goss. *Nutrition Against Aging*. New York: Bantam, 1983.

183. Wurtman, Judith J., Ph.D. *Managing Your Mind and Mood Through Food*. New York: Rawson Associates, 1986.

184. Zak, Victoria, Chris Carlin, M.S., R.D., and Peter Vash, M.D., M.P.H. *The Fat-to-Muscle Diet*. New York: G. P. Putnam's Sons, 1987.

Index